The Positive Thyroid Pregnancy Book

Your Essential Guide to Navigating Fertility, Pregnancy & Postpartum Wellness With Hypothyroidism and Hashimoto's

By Rachel Hill, The Invisible Hypothyroidism

First published in 2025. Copyright © Rachel Gask, 2025

Rachel Gask asserts the moral right to be identified as the author of this work, and to be identified as the author of this work in accordance with the Copyright, Designs and Patent Act 1988. All rights reserved.

No part of this book may be used or reproduced in any manner whatsoever, electronic or mechanical, including photocopying, recording or by any information storage or retrieval system, without written permission from the author, except in case of brief quotations embodied in critical articles and reviews.

No generative artificial intelligence (AI) was used in the writing of this work. The author expressly prohibits any entity from using either text or illustrations in this publication for the purpose of training AI technologies, including without limitation, technologies that are capable of generating works in the same style or genre as this publication. The author reserves all rights to license use of this work for generative AI training and development of machine learning language models.

Copies are available at special rates for bulk orders, please contact rachel@theinvisiblehypothyroidism.com.

Up to date contact information can be found at:
www.theinvisiblehypothyroidism.com

First Edition.
ISBN: 978-1-9160903-3-0

Praise for Rachel Hill and The Positive Thyroid Pregnancy Book

"For women with thyroid conditions, pregnancy can feel overwhelming—filled with uncertainty, conflicting advice, and concerns about how to best support both their health and their baby's development. The Positive Thyroid Pregnancy Book brings together the latest research and practical, compassionate guidance to help women optimize their thyroid health before, during, and after pregnancy.

If you've ever worried about how your thyroid will impact your fertility, pregnancy, or postpartum recovery, this book is a must-read. It provides the knowledge and confidence to take charge of your health and ensure the best possible start for your little one!"
- Izabella Wentz, PharmD, The Thyroid Pharmacist and #1 New York Times Bestselling Author of Hashimoto's Protocol.

"Rachel's book is exactly what thyroid patients need—practical wisdom that replaces fear with hope. It is a must for anyone navigating pregnancy with thyroid disease. I'll be recommending it to all my readers."
- Dr. Alan Christianson, New York Times bestselling author of The Thyroid Reset Diet.

"Rachel's compassionate guidance fills a critical gap, offering comfort, confidence, and crucial support to thyroid patients on the path to parenthood. This empowering and uplifting guide is one I wish had existed during my own pregnancy journey."
- Ginny Mahar, FMCHC, Hypothyroid Chef.

"Following your advice, I managed to get pregnant! Not sure how because I only had one natural period in 9 months but somehow fell pregnant! I feel your advice has helped, so thank you!"
- Instagram Follower.

"This book is very practical, informative & hopeful. Importantly it also fills a gap in the thyroid health world for patients looking to fall pregnant or who have already faced challenges in doing so. Rachel's conversational writing style is perfect for the deeply personal & often sensitive topic of pregnancy."
- Annabel Bateman, Author & Podcast Host of Let's Talk Thyroid.

"This book is an incredibly helpful and straightforward guide for women navigating pregnancy with Hashimoto's. It provides clear, actionable steps while diving into the necessary details, making it both easy to follow and thorough. I can't wait to recommend this to my own patients as they work towards fertility and managing their thyroid health. A must-read for any woman dealing with these challenges!"
- Victoria Gasparini, Naturopathic Medical Graduate, Founder of TheFedupThyroid, and Host of the Girls Gone Wellness Podcast.

Dedication

This book is dedicated to my two wonderful children, born in 2020 and 2022. Rainbow babies; I'm so lucky to be your mummy.

This book is also dedicated to the baby I never got to meet and the many others lost to thyroid patients around the world. We will not forget you.

Acknowledgements

My husband Adam, who continues to be my biggest cheerleader and believer in my mission with The Invisible Hypothyroidism. He's also the wonderful father of my two children and who has weathered the storms with me through a pregnancy loss and anxieties embarking on subsequent pregnancies, not knowing what may be in store. For holding my hand through the difficult appointments. For all the technical support you have provided in putting this book together. Thank you. You're my rock.

Deborah Panesar, who illustrated the book cover and had the wonderful concept of combining the thyroid symbol of a butterfly with a pregnancy test. Thank you for your creativity.

Most importantly, this book and any of my work as *The Invisible Hypothyroidism* would not be possible without the thousands of thyroid patients worldwide who continue to follow and support me across my website, social media channels and email newsletters. Thank you for sharing your experiences too. Our thyroid community is amazing.

Disclaimer (the boring legal stuff)

This book is compiled to provide information and education on health. It contains information that is intended to help the reader become a better-informed consumer of healthcare. Its publication is not intended to replace the relationship with your doctor or any other medical professional and their guidance. Neither the publisher, author, or anyone involved with making this book, mentioned or quoted in the book, takes responsibility for any consequences of any treatment, actions or application of any method by any person reading or following the information contained in this book.

Therefore, it is recommended that you consult with your physician regarding any drugs, supplements, diet changes or other treatments and therapies that may be beneficial to you. The reader should regularly consult a physician in matters relating to their health. Every effort has been made to ensure that this book is as complete and accurate as possible, however, there may be mistakes, both typographical and in content. This book contains information that should be assumed correct only up to the printing date.

Although the author has made every effort to ensure that the information in this book was correct at time of printing, the author does not assume and hereby disclaims any liability or responsibility to any party for any loss, damage, or disruption caused by errors or omissions, whether such errors or omissions result from negligence, accident, or any other cause.

About the Author

Rachel Hill is the highly ranked and multi-award winning thyroid patient advocate, certified patient leader, writer, speaker and author behind The Invisible Hypothyroidism.

Her books are bestselling and adored the world over by the thyroid patient community. Her thyroid advocacy work includes writing, public speaking, running online support spaces, appearing on radio, television and podcasts, as well as creating her popular social media content and email newsletters, all around thyroid awareness and advocacy.
She is well-recognised as a crucial contributor to the thyroid community and has received multiple awards and recognitions for her work and dedication, including a WEGO Health Award and Social Health Award.

Rachel lives in England with her husband Adam and two young sons, and can often be found cooking, baking, gardening, reading and juggling motherhood with the practices she knows are important for her thyroid health. She loves being in nature, walking, yoga and dance classes.

To keep up to date with Rachel, please visit her website TheInvisibleHypothyroidism.com, follow her on social media and sign up to her newsletter, where you will find she's collated all the must-know information for thyroid patients around the globe.

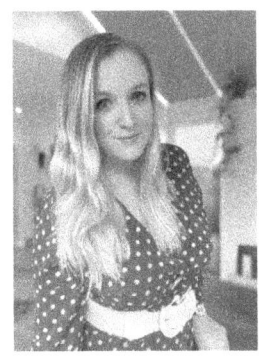

Contents

Preface i

Introduction... v

Part One: Optimising Your Fertility 7

Chapter 1: Your Thyroid Gland's Role in Fertility and Pregnancy... 9

Chapter 2: Making One of The Biggest Decisions of Your Life 25

Chapter 3: Optimising Fertility With Hypothyroidism......... 31

Part Two: Promoting a Healthy Pregnancy 91

Chapter 4: Being a Pregnant Thyroid Patient.........................95

Chapter 5: Exercising While Pregnant.................................. 125

Chapter 6: Your Healthcare Team in Pregnancy 133

Chapter 7: Rachel's Pregnancies (and how they were so different!).. 141

Chapter 8: Giving Birth 157

Part Three: Taking Care of Yourself During Postpartum and Parenting 163

Chapter 9: What Does Thyroid Health Look Like After Pregnancy? 165

Chapter 10: Postpartum Mental Health 181

Chapter 11: Breastfeeding With Hypothyroidism 187

Chapter 12: Parenting With Hypothyroidism 195

Extra Resources	209
A Letter To My 2020 Baby…	211
Tests You May Need and Where to Order Them	213
List of Thyroid (And Related) Events	215
Further Sources of Information	217
Index	223
Appendix (References)	229

Preface

Hi, I'm a thyroid patient advocate. I have hypothyroidism caused by Hashimoto's. I have also been pregnant three times. The first ended in a miscarriage, the second and third resulted in healthy, full-term babies.

(For simplicity in this book, when I mention 'my first pregnancy' and 'my second pregnancy' I am referring to the two pregnancies which resulted in the births of my children)

Before attempting to conceive, I was filled with anxiety whenever I thought about it. Anxiety whenever I looked ahead to hopefully having a family one day, yet I was still in a terrible place with thyroid symptoms taking control of my life. The kind of thoughts that entered my head included "How on Earth will I ever be able to look after a baby, when I can't even look after myself?" and "Will I even be able to have a child?". Especially since my thyroid condition sent my periods out of whack and I wasn't ovulating for years.

This book comes from a deeply personal need to provide the information not currently available out there. There is a huge lack of information surrounding thyroid disease and trying to conceive, yes, but an even bigger lack about navigating pregnancy and then not forgetting what comes after: the postpartum period and parenting. After all, your thyroid condition doesn't go away when you become a parent.

Furthermore, thyroid conditions often flare under stress, unpredictability and lack of sleep; three things I have learned come in abundance with that little bundle of joy!

THE POSITIVE THYROID PREGNANCY BOOK

When you turn to the internet to ask questions about trying to conceive or having a healthy pregnancy with thyroid disease, what you often find is anxiety-provoking. There is a lack of positive reassurance for thyroid patients. We are bombarded with articles, stories and rates of miscarriage, stillbirth, birth defects, the baby having congenital hypothyroidism or autism. It is easy to therefore assume that we are far more likely to have a tricky experience instead of the truth, that many of us *can* have healthy pregnancies and healthy babies when we have a thyroid disease diagnosis. We just need to know how.

This is my fourth book, following the overwhelming success of *Be Your Own Thyroid Advocate*, which started my journey as an author in 2018, *You, Me and Hypothyroidism* in 2019 and *Thyroid Superhero* in 2023. Much like my first book, I wanted to mesh both my personal experiences (of fertility, pregnancy, postpartum and parenting with thyroid disease), with the science, guidelines and in other words, *crucial information* my fellow thyroid patients also need, in order to navigate and feel supported through this life-changing time. Whilst pregnant with my first son in 2019, I felt the importance of writing this book deep in my bones. I was learning so much valuable information firsthand that I knew needed to be shared far and wide.

Following my miscarriage in 2018, I embarked on a fourteen month journey to optimise my health as much as possible before trying to conceive again. Even though my miscarriage was very early on, at around 6 weeks, and happened without complications (I did not need any medical interventions), it was still very painful to experience and process. I had yearned to be a mother for a long time. That baby was really wanted. Furthermore, it wasn't until I had birthed and held my first child in 2020 that I started to feel some healing from that experience.

Between 2018 and 2019, in order to increase my chances of a healthy pregnancy and baby at the end of it, I did a lot of research. I delved into books, website articles, guidelines, research, patient stories and more, to gather the best information I could. Thankfully, this chapter was followed by two healthy children, arriving in 2020 and 2022, though both pregnancies were very different experiences when it came to the management of my thyroid condition, as I'll share in this book!

Sharing online the information I felt to be crucial, I knew it needed a better, improved format: a book. Information around a topic like this is best delivered in a concise, easy to digest, all-in-one-place format. Not in fragments all over social media!

So, I started writing this book while still pregnant with my first child in 2019 and have (*very* slowly!) plugged away at it over the last five years or so because, consequently, becoming a parent to two little people has very quickly absorbed most of my time! I am confident that it has been worth the wait. I am very proud of it.

My hope for this book is that more thyroid patients will feel empowered to make the right decisions for them on their fertility and parenting journey. My hope is that less babies will be lost and that, maybe years from now, I will hear about the much-wanted babies this book helped to bring into the world.

I often wonder: if I had had the information contained in this book when I first started trying to conceive, would the baby I lost be here? Could my painful experience somehow benefit others, through this book, and save them from that heartbreak?

THE POSITIVE THYROID PREGNANCY BOOK

I am not a doctor, that is true, but I *am* a fellow thyroid patient living with this health condition and I know the ins and outs of that experience. I advocate for thyroid patients through authoring books, writing articles, creating social media content, running online spaces, writing regular newsletters, speaking at events, sitting on boards and so much more. My work has been recognised with multiple awards and accolades. However, none of this means as much to me as knowing I could save others the pain I experienced with my pregnancy loss.

Yes, my work as a leading patient advocate in the thyroid world (or, 'thyroidsphere', as I like to call it) began in 2015 with my own diagnosis of autoimmune hypothyroidism, but my learning is ongoing. I am constantly open to understanding more about this, and going through my own pregnancy and fertility journey opened up my eyes to the lack of information available about this in an easily accessible format.

So, although it has been a very unpleasant journey at times, it has led me to this point today and that has to mean something positive.

I'm so excited to have you here.

Rachel Hill, The Invisible Hypothyroidism

Introduction

The Positive Thyroid Pregnancy Book is, I hope, a refreshing, uplifting and helpful tool in your own journey to parenthood. Wherever you may be in that.

Some will be picking up this book as they think about wanting to conceive one day in the future. Others will be trying to conceive already and are perhaps having a hard time falling pregnant or staying pregnant. Others may already be pregnant and are looking for guidance on supporting that pregnancy and their body after birth. Wherever you join us from, welcome.

My fourth book remains true to the style of writing you may already know me for; personal, honest and non-technical. There are many great books on thyroid disease, written by many great thyroid experts. However, my style of writing can feel different to others in the thyroidsphere, as I am not writing with a medical degree nor PhD. I'm a thyroid patient sharing hers and others' firsthand experiences in the hopes of making change to how we're perceived and treated in this world. People with thyroid disease do not get an easy ride!

As well as *my own* experiences with fertility, pregnancy, postpartum and parenting being covered in this book, I have also drawn in all the guidelines and research others need in order to feel clued-up, too.

Some of the information shared in this book is from a functional medicine perspective, so it's worth keeping in mind that your mainstream medicine doctor may not be aware of it all. They may not even support it. However, I hope you will feel your own confidence to advocate for yourself (and any child you may go on to grow and carry) build and uplift you.

Because this is the truth: when you fall pregnant or are wishing to, you are no longer just advocating for yourself. You are also advocating for the health of your unborn child.

Anyone wishing to go through pregnancy should feel empowered. They should know the incredible things that their body can do. They should know their rights and feel they can choose their care as an informed person. The purpose of this book is to do all of this.

Throughout my two successful pregnancies, I saw both a GP on the NHS here in the UK and a private GP, who currently prescribes my thyroid medication and is based in London. I also saw midwives, NHS endocrinologists and obstetricians, and I will cover where all of these practitioners fit in the larger picture in this book, as well as perhaps where some may be more or less helpful than others.

You will find that this book is split into the three key parts of your journey to parenthood: Fertility, Pregnancy and Postpartum & Parenting. Depending on where you are in your journey, you may wish to jump to a particular section, but if you are yet to be pregnant (or a few months in, past the riskiest time for pregnancy loss, the first trimester), you will get the most out of it by reading it from start to finish. Grab some pens and highlighters and make notes as you go along. Underline or highlight sections that apply to you and things you wish to explore or implement off the back of it. I did this with all of my pregnancy and parenting books and it made it so much easier to refer back to. Your journey to parenthood is unique and individual to you. Make this book the same and you'll get the most out of it. Highlighter at the ready? Let's go!

Part One: Optimising Your Fertility

Chapter 1: Your Thyroid Gland's Role in Fertility and Pregnancy

To understand what we can do to promote a healthy conception and pregnancy with thyroid disease, it is first important to understand what the thyroid gland is and how it works.

What is Hypothyroidism?

Hypothyroidism, also called an underactive thyroid or referred to as thyroid disease, is a condition where the thyroid, a butterfly-shaped gland in the neck, does not create enough thyroid hormone. The five hormones a healthy thyroid produces are: T1, T2, T3, T4 and Calcitonin. The most important are T3 and T4, with T3 being the most active.

These hormones are needed for every process, every cell and every function in the body, so when they are too low, as is the case with hypothyroidism, the effects can be far-reaching.

This can include:

- Metabolic function
- Sensitivity to heat
- Cold intolerance
- Muscle or joint aches and pains, cramps and weakness
- Fatigue
- Nutrient deficiencies
- Weight gain and inability to lose weight
- Constipation

- Depression, anxiety and other mental health difficulties
- Slow movements, speech and thoughts
- Itchy and sore scalp
- Poor appetite
- Dry and tight feeling skin
- Brittle hair and nails
- Loss of libido (sex drive)
- Pain, numbness or a tingling sensation in hands/fingers
- Numbness in limbs
- Menstrual complaints
- Brain fog, confusion and memory problems
- Migraines
- Hoarse voice
- A puffy-looking face (called 'moon face')
- Thinned or partly missing eyebrows
- Hearing loss
- Poor stamina
- Feeling weak
- The need to nap more than others
- Long recovery period after activity
- Inability to exercise, or withstand certain exercises
- Diagnosis of Chronic Fatigue Syndrome
- Feeling very emotional
- Poor circulation
- High or rising cholesterol
- Acid reflux
- IBS
- Hair loss
- Easy bruising
- Swollen legs that impede walking
- Shin splints
- Difficulty standing on feet
- Fertility issues

Many people find that they have their own combination of this long list of symptoms or experience symptoms not included here. In fact, this list is by no means exhaustive; I'm always hearing about new symptoms. Conditions such as hypothyroidism are often experienced on a scale, with some people having no symptoms at all, some having a few mild symptoms, and others experiencing many severe symptoms, to the point of it impacting their work life, social life, relationships and more.

The main purpose of thyroid hormone is to ensure that the metabolism is running correctly, with the metabolism's job being to produce heat and fuel. Heat to keep us warm and fuel to give us energy. If we do not have enough thyroid hormone, our metabolism cannot work properly and provide us with adequate heat and fuel. Therefore, people with hypothyroidism often have a slow metabolism and symptoms such as cold intolerance (from the lack of heat made) and extreme tiredness and weight gain (from the lack of calories burned to make energy). Hypothyroidism is classed as a chronic health condition or 'chronic illness' because of its tendency to be with us for the rest of our lives.

Hypothyroidism affects us all slightly differently, as some people report taking their medication each day and feeling fine, whereas others report that their medication does not help them, or that it did at one time, but not anymore.

Ultimately, once thyroid hormone levels are optimised (defined in Chapter 3) and the thyroid condition is being optimally addressed, most symptoms should start to disappear, but support for other possible problems like autoimmune disease (Hashimoto's), vitamin deficiencies and adrenal dysfunction for example, will need to be in place until they are addressed, too. Ongoing monitoring to maintain optimal thyroid hormone levels is important, which should also help keep vitamin levels and adrenal health in check, too, along with any other associated conditions, symptoms and complaints.

If you are on thyroid medication and still feel unwell, then you may not be converting T4 (stored thyroid hormone) into adequate amounts of T3 (active thyroid hormone), which is needed in order for you to feel well. This is the main reason why so many people with hypothyroidism and on medication for it still feel unwell.

Although we have more T4 than T3 in our bodies, T3 is the most active and most useful thyroid hormone. It is what impacts how we feel. T4 is around 90% of what the thyroid gland produces, with around 9% being T3. Enough levels of both are needed to help us feel well and carry out all our usual bodily functions and processes. If you are on T4-only medication such as Levothyroxine or Synthroid, then the T4 must convert to enough T3 to correct the hypothyroidism and feel well.

An inability to properly convert T4 to T3 is common among thyroid patients and can result in a fluctuating TSH, or a TSH that is 'in range' and a low Free T3 level. This is why it is so important to have the full thyroid panel tested and not just TSH.

The full panel consists of:

- TSH
- Free T3
- Free T4
- Thyroid Peroxidase Antibodies
- Thyroglobulin Antibodies

If you do not already, please obtain and keep copies of all your test results so you can see for yourself *what* exactly is being tested and whether the results are in fact optimised (explained in the next chapter). This cannot be refused as they are *your* medical records.

Many people on thyroid hormone replacement medications such as Synthroid or Levothyroxine have a normal TSH level, yet when they check their Free T3 and Free T4 levels, they see that the T4 from their thyroid medication is not converting to adequate levels of T3.

This may be caused by a deficiency in an enzyme called iodothyronine deiodinase, if you have the Deiodinase 2 (DIO2) gene variant. However, many of us won't know this! The DIO2 gene was researched in 2009 and the results were published in a paper titled *"Common Variation in the DIO2 Gene Predicts Baseline Psychological Well-Being and Response to Combination Thyroxine plus Triiodothyronine Therapy in Hypothyroid Patients."*

The DIO2 gene activates the active thyroid hormone T3. The researchers found that a small change in this gene could mean that thyroid patients have ongoing symptoms on T4-only medicines such as Levothyroxine.

Patients in this study were given Levothyroxine for a set period and then combination treatment of both Levothyroxine and liothyronine (synthetic T3). The patients who had normal genes did not feel any different on the combination treatment, but those who had the DIO2 gene felt better on combination treatment.[1]

The enzyme iodothyronine deiodinase is important in the activation and deactivation of thyroid hormones, as T4 is converted into T3 by deiodinase activity. A problem with this can therefore cause conversion issues, where TSH may look 'fine', as well as the Free T4 level, but with a low Free T3 and continued hypothyroid symptoms and development of other health conditions. Low or deficient levels of trace minerals Selenium and Zinc can also cause conversion issues since this process requires these nutrients. Supplementing these may therefore help with conversion, but the vast majority are likely to have the DIO2 gene which can only be addressed with direct T3 medication.

The gut assists in converting T4 to T3, which requires an enzyme called intestinal sulfatase. However, this enzyme comes from healthy gut bacteria, therefore, an unhealthy gut can lead to a lack of this important enzyme and thus, contribute to poor T4 to T3 conversion. Intestinal dysbiosis is an imbalance between pathogenic and beneficial bacteria in the gut, which can significantly reduce thyroid hormone conversion. This is one reason why people with poor gut health may have thyroid symptoms but 'normal' TSH test results. Chapter 3 talks about optimising your gut health.

If you are one of the many who still feel unwell on synthetic T4-only medications such as Levothyroxine and Synthroid, due to not converting enough T3, then adding in direct T3 is the way to go, for your overall health, quality of life, but also your fertility and beyond. This is explained further in Chapter 3.

Other names for hypothyroidism include *an underactive thyroid, low thyroid*, the general terms *thyroid disease and thyroid disorder, congenital hypothyroidism* if it has existed since birth, and *autoimmune hypothyroidism* if it is caused by Hashimoto's Thyroiditis.

What is 'Borderline' or 'Subclinical' Hypothyroidism?

I was one of the many people diagnosed with 'subclinical hypothyroidism'. Also called 'borderline hypothyroidism', it refers to test results just outside or just within normal reference limits.

An example of subclinical hypothyroidism could be a TSH test result of 5 on a range of 1-4. However, it is important to keep in mind that lab ranges differ from lab to lab and country to country. The inconsistency on what constitutes subclinical hypothyroidism can be wild, therefore, we must go by our own test results and ranges.

Many people are told that their thyroid levels are 'subclinically hypothyroid' and not yet 'bad enough' for treatment, even though they are nowhere near the optimal TSH level of 2.5 or below, which is why they're likely having ongoing thyroid symptoms.

Another problem that the term 'subclinical hypothyroidism' creates is that many doctors go by TSH levels alone for a thyroid condition diagnosis, and TSH is a pituitary hormone. So, whilst our TSH level may only be 'mildly' borderline, actual thyroid hormone levels Free T3 and Free T4 could be much lower and it also does not take into account thyroid antibodies.

If you're testing positive for thyroid peroxidase antibodies and thyroglobulin antibodies, which check for Hashimoto's, then your thyroid hormone levels are pretty much guaranteed to continue worsening with time, unless the antibodies are addressed. Ways to reduce these antibodies may include taking thyroid medication as well as tackling other lifestyle areas, but do you have the energy to implement these without treatment for your 'mild hypothyroidism' if it's causing you fatigue? It's a hard cycle and we need to start somewhere.

Many of us see the effects of a high TSH differently. For example, the range my doctor used was 0.5-5, and I felt very, very ill with a TSH of 9, which he described as 'mildly borderline'. Others have told me that they got to a TSH of 4, 50 or 100 before feeling unwell. Therefore, we should be treated individually and more than TSH should be checked.

Does everyone who is subclinically hypothyroid need thyroid hormone replacement medication? Not necessarily. However, women with subclinical hypothyroidism should be given extra consideration when trying to conceive or are pregnant, as we'll discuss some more later on.

Hashimoto's

You may be reading this book right now and have no idea that you even have this autoimmune disease. You may have never been tested but knowing whether Hashimoto's Thyroiditis is the cause for your hypothyroidism or underactive thyroid is beneficial in your treatment and efforts to make progress in how you feel, as well as your journey to parenthood.

Hashimoto's is an autoimmune disease that causes the body to attack and destroy its own thyroid gland, leading to hypothyroidism as the thyroid begins to dysfunction (lose ability to produce as much thyroid hormone as it should) from the damage caused. As time goes by, if this autoimmune disease is not well controlled, your body continues to destroy the thyroid, causing a greater loss of function, which can lead to test results getting gradually worse, a diagnosis of hypothyroidism, followed by increases in thyroid medication dosage and worsening symptoms.

To know if you have Hashimoto's, you need two tests running: TPOAB (Thyroid Peroxidase Antibodies) and TGAB (Thyroglobulin Antibodies). You preferably need both testing, as just the one test is not accurate enough to be sure. One could have results 'in range', while the other not.

Having Hashimoto's will usually show as TPOAB and TGAB test results being above range, but did you know that you can still have Hashimoto's without the positive antibodies? Yes, negative antibodies do not necessarily mean that you don't have the autoimmune condition.

We know that Hashimoto's is responsible for around 90% of cases of hypothyroidism, so this leaves up to 10% having Hashimoto's but coming back negative on antibody tests. This can be due to a number of reasons, such as antibody numbers moving up and down and catching the lower number when you test, or certain lifestyle interventions such as Selenium and Vitamin D supplementation, gluten and dairy-free diets lowering antibodies in some people, or your overall immune system being so weak that you do not produce enough of the antibodies, as suggested by thyroid expert Dr Datis Kharrazian.[2]

It is worth knowing that you could see variations in your thyroid antibody and TSH results each time you test, as they swing up and down. This is a common sign of Hashimoto's, as ongoing destruction of your thyroid gland causes sudden surges of thyroid hormone to be released into the blood.

It is common for doctors to refuse to test thyroid antibodies, as they often do not see the importance of knowing whether your hypothyroidism is autoimmune, because for many doctors, they're only going to give you the standard T4-only medication whether you have Hashimoto's or not. In their eyes, it does not change your treatment. However, this is where I disagree. Whether you have Hashimoto's, an autoimmune condition, matters and it matters especially when it comes to your fertility and pregnancy.

You could choose to go private to have these tests run if your doctor refuses or order them yourself online. More and more people are doing this as it has become a lot more accessible in recent years.[3]

If you have Hashimoto's, then you can look at calming down the attack on your thyroid gland and lowering those high antibody levels. By doing this, it is believed that the attack against your thyroid is slowed down or halted, meaning that symptoms disappear and recovery can begin. When it comes to fertility and pregnancy, reduced thyroid antibody levels are linked with better outcomes. I will cover all this in this book!

If Hashimoto's is the cause for around 90% of the cases of hypothyroidism, what causes the other 10%?

Surgery

Surgery to remove the thyroid gland (a thyroidectomy) will lead to hypothyroidism. If only part of the thyroid is removed, what is remaining may be able to produce enough thyroid hormone alone, but commonly does not, so thyroid hormone replacement medication is required to replace the hormones that are missing. Surgery to remove the thyroid gland may be performed for thyroid cancer, overactive thyroid disease such as Graves' Disease, hyperthyroidism and Hashitoxicosis.

RAI

Radioactive Iodine Treatment, also often called Radioactive Iodine Therapy, RAI, RI or remnant ablation, is an effective way to kill off thyroid tissue. It can be used on its own or in conjunction with a thyroidectomy.

Usually taken as a 'drink' or tablet, radioactive Iodine is taken up by the thyroid and destroys thyroid cells. This effectively reduces the amount of thyroid hormone made by the gland and usually, to the point of disabling it altogether.

A treatment often used for hyperthyroidism (an overactive thyroid), RAI often results in hypothyroidism, where the thyroid is permanently disabled from working at all or working less than it used to.

Genetics

Sometimes, it's just in your genes. The thyroid gland may not correctly develop during utero or at birth, meaning that it is absent or underdeveloped. This can lead to someone being born with congenital hypothyroidism. For some babies, their thyroid gland does not form in its normal position in the neck.

The thyroid gland may also start to falter later on in life, which is more common. Dr Barry Durrant-Peatfield describes it as being 'programmed to fail', in his book *Your Thyroid and how to keep it healthy.. The Great Thyroid Scandal and How to Survive it.* He is essentially saying that your thyroid going under active was a bit of a ticking time-bomb. It was always going to fail due to genes you have inherited, but we do not always know when, although if it runs in your family, you may have noticed a pattern. For example, many families see women develop a thyroid condition at the same sort of age or time in their life, such as in puberty, postpartum or during the menopause.

It also appears that having Down Syndrome increases the risk of having hypothyroidism.

Deficiencies

Deficiencies in certain nutrients can also lead to hypothyroidism. Iodine deficiency is well-recognised, as adequate Iodine is needed for proper thyroid function. Adequate Selenium levels are another important part of thyroid function.

The Contraceptive Pill

Many functional medicine practitioners state that too much oestrogen, often caused by the contraceptive pill or birth control pill, can lead to hypothyroidism. Contraceptive pills can also deplete vitamins and nutrients, leading to deficiencies that increase thyroid hormone binding meaning that less is available for use by cells. Excess oestrogen can also affect how much thyroid hormone is used by the body.

Adrenal Dysfunction

A failing thyroid gland can cause the adrenals to become stressed and fatigued, but what if you have adrenal dysfunction first, that leads to hypothyroidism? Another possible cause or contributing factor. We cover the role of the adrenal glands further on in this book.

Trauma

Direct damage such as whiplash, injury to the throat or hitting your chin on the dashboard in a car accident can understandably lead to a damaged thyroid gland.

Central Hypothyroidism

Although rare, if something is wrong with the pituitary gland, this can interfere with the production of thyroid hormones. The pituitary gland produces TSH, which tells the thyroid how much hormone it should make and release. If something is wrong with the pituitary gland, then thyroid hormone production and release will be affected, causing hypothyroidism.

A similar problem can be of the hypothalamus too. Although rare as well, hypothyroidism can occur if the hypothalamus, situated in the brain, does not produce enough TRH, which tells the pituitary to release TSH.

What Caused Yours?

It is believed that those of us carrying the genetic makeup to develop a thyroid issue trigger the condition by switching it 'on'. It is most often a combination of genetic susceptibility plus environmental triggers, such as hormonal changes, excess Iodine, viruses and stress, which lead to the onset of a thyroid condition.

If something causes a big enough stress to the body, it can be a contributing trigger. There is no one cause or trigger for everyone, and what's more, we can all experience a different combination of unfortunate things that all contribute towards triggering the onset of a thyroid condition.

How Your Thyroid Impacts Your Fertility

Thyroid function and fertility are closely linked. Abnormal thyroid hormone levels in women can lead to miscarriage, pre-eclampsia, depression and anxiety during and after pregnancy, low birth weight, admission to NICU, anaemia, stillbirth and, in pregnancy, the baby being born with congenital hypothyroidism. For men with hypothyroidism, they can experience erectile dysfunction, infertility issues, low testosterone levels and lowered sperm mobility. Yes, fertility in both women and men can be impacted by a thyroid condition, yet many doctors do not think to check thyroid hormone levels in relation to fertility.

Thyroid hormones directly affect the uterine lining, which can cause infertility or miscarriages to occur when they are abnormal. As well as complications during pregnancy, some women with low thyroid levels may struggle to fall pregnant at all. Hormones TSH (thyroid stimulating hormone) and TRH (thyrotropin-releasing hormone) are increased when thyroid hormones such as Free T3 and Free T4 fall too low. TRH stimulates the pituitary gland to release TSH, which then instructs the thyroid gland to release more thyroid hormones T3 and T4.

Infertility can therefore occur when TRH, which is also responsible for stimulating the pituitary gland to release prolactin, causes the increased prolactin to interfere with the ovulation process, when thyroid hormones are low. The increased prolactin levels can prevent the ovaries from releasing an egg each month, which makes it impossible to conceive. Therefore, ensuring your thyroid levels are optimal is crucial when wanting to fall pregnant. For women with a known thyroid condition, it is not recommended to try conceiving unless they know their thyroid levels are optimised. Not doing so risks pregnancy loss and complications.

Additionally, if you have the autoimmune version of hypothyroidism, Hashimoto's, you'll want to keep a check on adequately treating the antibodies too, since some experts state that thyroid antibodies cross the human placenta and could attack the growing baby's thyroid gland. Research has also shown that high levels of Thyroid Peroxidase Antibodies increase the risk of premature births, so keeping Hashimoto's well controlled can be helpful.[4]

If you have been told that you are 'subclinical' or 'borderline' hypothyroid, your doctor may wish to start you on thyroid medication or increase it so that you're well within range to improve chances of conception and reduce the risk of miscarriage. The risk of miscarriage is higher in women with subclinical hypothyroidism, compared to women with normal thyroid function (euthyroidism).[5]

A study also found that among women with diminished ovarian reserve or unexplained infertility, low Free T3 levels and positive thyroid antibodies (TPOAB) are associated with low antral follicle count.[6]

In the first trimester of pregnancy, the foetus relies completely on the mother to provide the thyroid hormones for its development. For someone with a perfectly healthy thyroid gland and function, their body is able to meet that extra demand rather easily, but in a woman with hypothyroidism and/or Hashimoto's, her body is often not as able to. This is why the management of a thyroid condition during pregnancy is so important.

Bearing all of this in mind, this book will look at how we can work towards a well-managed thyroid condition, including your thyroid hormone levels and thyroid antibody levels, so that you can optimise your chances of a healthy pregnancy and baby at the end of it.

End of Chapter Checklist:

- ☐ I have a good understanding of what my thyroid gland is and why it is important.
- ☐ I have a good understanding of the symptoms of hypothyroidism and Hashimoto's.
- ☐ I have a good understanding of what my thyroid disease diagnosis is, and if I do not, I have made a note to confirm with my doctor (e.g. if it is hypothyroidism, Hashimoto's).

Chapter 2: Making One of The Biggest Decisions of Your Life

Many couples are excited at the prospect of starting or growing a family, but for those with hypothyroidism, there can be an added layer of worry and complication. Not only does having hypothyroidism increase the chances of pregnancy complications such as miscarriage, pre-eclampsia, anaemia, stillbirth and the baby being born with congenital hypothyroidism, but a thyroid patient's health during pregnancy and after birth can also be quite uncertain.

So how do you know if you're ready? It's such a personal decision that must take into account *your* family life, support available, financial situation as well as your health situation.

I know that for me, I didn't want to start a family until my health was in the best place I felt it could be, so that the chances of losing another pregnancy were reduced, but also so that my body could get through pregnancy as easily as possible, and still be standing after birth, when I knew a lot would be demanded from it. I wanted to be an active, involved and happy parent, after all.

My husband and I knew that there was never going to be a 'perfect' time to start a family. Work, my thyroid condition, house redecorating, travel, responsibilities and commitments, life events and so much more would always be around to some extent, so we went with a 'good time to have a baby' instead of waiting for the 'perfect time'.

To us, this looked like my health being stable (hypothyroidism well-controlled and Hashimoto's in remission), financially stable, at a point in our careers that meant we could pause or make sacrifices for a year or two (or even longer) and, for me, with age on my side if possible. After all, optimal fertility occurs for most women in their twenties.

Having been together since we were teenagers, we had originally planned to start a family when we turned 30, but this was before my thyroid condition struck in my early twenties. After having symptoms throughout my teen years, I was finally diagnosed with thyroid disease at 21-years-old and was in my mid-20's by the time it was well-managed and in remission. I would have periods of it flaring up again before resettling and this is when we decided: we would enjoy my current period of stable health for a year or so before attempting to conceive. I didn't want to bank on the fact that my health would be in a stable enough place in another five years or so when I hit that 30 years of age target we originally threw out there, and my husband agreed. So, we brought our plans to start a family forward.

We had been together for ten years by this time, were financially stable and all other criteria for us lined up, so we decided to go for it. And what you're reading in this book is what happened from that point onwards.

I am very happy with our decision to have our first child when I was 26 (and a half!) and our second at 28 (and three quarters!). While, yes, we were younger than some of our friends to start a family, it was what felt right *for us* and worked *for us*. We capitalised on my health being in the right place, but those other things on the criteria list were met too. This will not be the case for everyone, of course. We're all on different paths. Now in my thirties with two young children to look after, I wonder just how much more tired I would be starting a family now, and if my thyroid health would be as well-managed as it is now. I feel that having my first child in my mid-twenties was 100% the right choice for me. Will it be for everyone? Of course not! But I'm sharing this to encourage you to take a deep dive into *your* own needs and criteria. It's OK for plans to change if that's what makes sense for you. This can also work the other way, with some people moving their timeline back for other sensible reasons.

Do what is right for you and your situation. Do you have some conditions you want to meet before starting a family? Financial, work or other commitments? List them and have a serious and lengthy conversation with those who will be directly involved in raising a child with you.

Here are some of the most common concerns when deciding if the time is 'right'.

That you may struggle to fall pregnant.

Many of us with thyroid issues experience wonky menstrual cycles. You know the ones; irregular, all over the place and not so predictable. Periods like this may make it harder to fall pregnant (explained why in Chapter 3).

A lot of us are told that having a thyroid condition makes it harder to conceive, and while this can also be true, it's not definite for everyone. Plenty manage to fall pregnant easily, but it is still a valid concern.

When you have this concern, it may make you consider the timeline for starting a family or having another child.

That you'll experience more flares.

It is reasonable to expect an increase in thyroid flare days when pregnant and this can be hard to plan for, especially with work to maintain too.

When you have this concern, it can be difficult to know if you are at a place in your life where extra flare days in pregnancy can be worked around. If you are just starting in your career, it may feel too disruptive.

That you'll experience a loss.

A pregnancy loss, called a miscarriage before 20 weeks, is estimated to affect around 1 in 8 known pregnancies. However, the actual number is likely to be quite a bit higher if you include the miscarriages that happen very early on, before many people realise they're even pregnant.

Having a thyroid condition does increase this chance, but for the most part, only if your thyroid hormone levels and/or thyroid antibody levels are abnormal.

Having this concern is absolutely valid. It was a concern I had and unfortunately came true for me in 2018. I was terrified of it happening again. Although the information contained in this book cannot guarantee an avoidance of this for you, it does provide you with areas that hopefully you can feel more in control of and reduce those chances.

Another reason we started a family a few years earlier than planned was because I felt concerned about a miscarriage or *recurrent* miscarriages, so I wanted to factor in time to recover from them and how this may impact my thyroid health and leave me with even less time to start and grow a family.

Conclusion

When we take the above points into account, it may impact how we decide if 'now' is the right time, or whether these concerns need consideration first. Only you can figure that out.

You may also be reading this book after having a child or multiple children previously and now wanting another but your health being in a different place this time around, due to thyroid issues. It is worth keeping in mind that health outcomes for both mother and baby are best when a woman waits at least 18 months between the birth of one baby and conceiving another. Your body needs time to recover from the pregnancy, birth and postpartum stages it has already endured, including the adrenal impacts of this and the depletion of key nutrients. Give your body time to rebuild between pregnancies wherever possible, to increase your chances of an easier conception, healthier pregnancy, smoother birth and postpartum stage.

End of Chapter Checklist:

- ☐ I have talked through logistics of impacts to my thyroid condition with those I will need support from.
- ☐ I have considered what any flare days may look like while I am pregnant / parenting.
- ☐ It may not feel like the 'perfect' time to have a baby, but I feel it is a good time.
- ☐ I have considered whether I need mental health support while I am trying to conceive (such as from a counsellor or therapist).

Chapter 3: Optimising Fertility With Hypothyroidism

I fell pregnant immediately after trying to conceive in 2018, however, this pregnancy ended in an early miscarriage.

Before this, I had done *some* reading and research, but after the miscarriage, I decided that I wanted to delve into it even more so. In the fourteen months between the miscarriage and attempting to conceive again, I did everything in my power to put my health in the best place possible so as to try and avoid another pregnancy loss. This is what I am going to share in this chapter.

Thankfully, when I tried to conceive again fourteen months after the miscarriage, in 2019, and with my health in the best place it had ever been, I fell pregnant immediately once more and this time it stuck. In 2020 I welcomed my healthy baby.

When I wanted to try and conceive again in 2021, eighteen months after the birth of my first child, I fell pregnant immediately once more and I truly believe that revisiting the below areas again, optimised chances for me.

Everything mentioned in this chapter was pulled from a lot of researching and speaking with medical professionals in regards to thyroid disease and pregnancy. I hope it helps you as much as it did me.

It is also important to say that we do not always know the reason behind a miscarriage. However, preparing your body as much as possible can certainly help to optimise the chances of a healthy conception with thyroid disease.

As I often say, every person is unique and individual, and so our needs and requirements can be unique to us as well. I have detailed below what I personally did to get my health in the best place possible before I tried to conceive again, however, some of these may not apply to you. This is a big chapter because it needed to be. Don't worry, I've included the end of chapter checklist for you!

Step 1: Optimise Thyroid Hormone Levels

The first step to optimising fertility with hypothyroidism is to check that our thyroid hormone levels are optimal. Please note how I said 'optimal' and not just 'in range'. There is a difference!

Thyroid hormones directly affect the uterine lining, causing infertility or miscarriages to occur when they are abnormal. As well as complications during pregnancy, some women with low thyroid levels will struggle to fall pregnant at all.

A recent study found that among women with diminished ovarian reserve or unexplained infertility, low Free T3 levels and positive thyroid antibodies (TPOAB) are associated with low antral follicle count.[7]

Ensuring you are not only having the full thyroid panel tested (not just TSH), as well as then using these to optimise your thyroid treatment, is perhaps the most important thing you can do when you have a thyroid condition and want to conceive. It should certainly be your first step and something to discuss with your doctor in detail.

What Are Optimal Thyroid Levels?

When your doctor runs a test and you receive the results, your levels will either fall inside or outside of a given range. Ranges are stated in brackets beside the test result.

However, as thyroid patients, it is important that we advocate for ourselves when it comes to *where* in range they fall. After all, it is not just about falling within the range, we are looking for something more specific. 'Optimal levels' refer to a more specific section *within* the given range.

You'll find that many thyroid advocacies and progressive medical practitioners agree that when testing a thyroid panel (or "Thyroid Function Test"), optimal levels are:

- TSH less than 2.5 (and not below the bottom of the reference range)
- Free T3 around the top quarter of the given range
- Free T4 around mid-range
- Antibodies as low as possible / within the normal range

These optimal areas within the given range are where a lot of thyroid patients say they feel most well and their fertility is best supported. These optimal points are more specific than just falling within the very wide reference range.

For example, optimal levels could be: a TSH of 1.5, a Free T3 of 17.5 on a range of 10-20 and Free T4 at 15 on a range of 10-20. (please note: this is just an example – you must go by the lab ranges specific to you and included with *your* test results)

For you personally, you may feel best somewhere else within range, but you should try to find out and maintain levels at what you feel best at. This is the definition of optimising your thyroid treatment. Get a copy of your test results (they can't be withheld) and check for yourself. It feels very empowering!

As of September 2024, NICE Guidelines state:

"If symptoms of hypothyroidism persist, consider adjusting the dose of LT4 further to achieve optimal wellbeing, taking care to avoid overtreatment. This is based on the fact that some people may still have troublesome symptoms even with TSH levels in the reference range, and changes in LT4 dose may improve symptoms for some people." [8]

Backing up the need for optimal T4 levels, not just an in-range TSH level.

The British Thyroid Foundation (BTF) state:

"Experts in the field recommend that if you are on Levothyroxine the TSH level should ideally be kept in the lower half of the reference range before pregnancy as this has been associated with a lower risk of miscarriage." [9]

For thyroid patients on T3 containing thyroid medication, such as T3 synthetic Liothyronine or natural desiccated thyroid medications, it is worth noting that the higher amount of T3 in these (compared to the ratio of T4 to T3 in a human thyroid gland) may have a suppressive effect on TSH. Therefore, your TSH may be suppressed (below the bottom of the range), yet your Free T3 and Free T4 remain within range and not close to overmedication or hyperthyroidism.[10]

Thyroid patients who have had a thyroidectomy may notice that in order to raise their Free T3 and T4 to optimal, their TSH needs to be suppressed too.[11]

Furthermore, for those who have had thyroid cancer, doctors may suppress TSH with thyroid medication, to reduce the chances of cancer reoccurring, deciding that the benefits outweigh the risks.

In 2002, the National Academy of Clinical Biochemistry (NACB) issued new guidelines for the diagnosis and monitoring of thyroid disease, which reported that the TSH reference range was too wide and actually included people with thyroid disease, thus making it inaccurate.

When more sensitive screening was done, which excluded people with thyroid disease, 95% of the population tested had a TSH level between 0.4 and 2.5. As a result, the NACB recommended reducing the reference range to those levels.[12]

Based on the NACB's findings, in January 2003, just a few months later, the AACE (American Association of Clinical Endocrinologists) made this announcement:

"Until November 2002, doctors had relied on a normal TSH level ranging from 0.5 to 5 to diagnose and treat patients with a thyroid disorder who tested outside the boundaries of that range. Now AACE encourages doctors to consider treatment for patients who test outside the boundaries of a narrower margin based on a target TSH level of 0.3 to 3. AACE believes the new range will result in proper diagnosis for millions of Americans who suffer from a mild thyroid disorder, but have gone untreated until now."

Furthermore, the third National Health and Nutrition Examination Survey (NHANES III) screened 17,353 subjects from 1988 to 1994 and excluded those with diseases or factors known to affect thyroid function too. In the resultant 'normal' population of 13,344 subjects, 95% had TSH levels that fell between 0.3 and 2.5, which is almost identical to the findings of the NACB above, again, backing up a TSH below 2.5.[13]

Regarding aiming for a Free T3 higher in range, a 2018 study reported that:

"Hypothyroid symptom relief was associated with both a T4 dose giving TSH-suppression below the lower reference limit and FT3 elevated further into the upper half of its reference range." [14]

and

"Residual hypothyroid complaints in LT4-treated patients are specifically related to low FT3 concentrations. This supports an important role of FT3 for clinical decision making on dose adequacy, particularly in symptomatic athyreotic patients."

A study titled The Definition of Optimal Metabolism and its association with large reductions in chronic diseases also said:

"Very simply, cells require an optimal amount of T3, the main thyroid hormone for ideal performance… Optimal Metabolism is measurable and specifically defined by the FT3 (free T3) in the upper 20% of the normal range… Being in the Optimal Range predictably coincides with substantial reductions in chronic diseases including Subclinical Hypothyroidism and other low T3 states." [15]

It is important to understand that different labs and doctors use different ranges, so you must interpret your results individually; don't compare them to anyone else's. You must use your lab's reference ranges.

Your doctor should be open to adjusting your dose to move you within the reference range. This really isn't an unreasonable request, but some persuading, listing your ongoing symptoms, may be needed. So go in prepared and be ready to see a different doctor or OBGYN if the first is not openminded.

What do you do if you find that your current thyroid medication is not optimising all thyroid levels? It is at this point that you may need to explore other options. T4-only thyroid medications in particular, such as Levothyroxine and Synthroid, can leave Free T3 levels below optimal, due to conversion issues, as explained in Chapter 1.

When I miscarried, I found out that my Free T4 had dropped to below range and I will always wonder if this was the cause or a contributing factor to the pregnancy loss. It certainly wasn't supportive, especially as demand for T4 increases as soon as you become pregnant. If you fall pregnant with levels already too low, it can be a recipe for heartache. So please do have the full set of thyroid tests checked and optimised before attempting to fall pregnant. I regret not doing this.

Thyroid medication options range from T4-only synthetics to T3-only synthetics, to NDT's and compounded NDT, or combining a couple of these. For example, some thyroid patients take synthetic T3 and synthetic T4 together, or synthetic T4 with NDT.

A note on T3 medications in pregnancy: many mainstream doctors are not comfortable prescribing and dosing them in pregnancy. NDT's such as Armour Thyroid and synthetic T3 are not as widely used or widely recommended for pregnancy. Being on T3-only medication (Cytomel, Liothyronine) during pregnancy is not usually recommended because of a lack of T4 for the foetus, which is the only thyroid hormone that crosses the placenta during development. Whether a doctor keeps you on these types of medications is up to their discretion.

Research has not yet been conducted on pregnant women taking anything other than T4-only medications in pregnancy, therefore many doctors are not comfortable with managing a pregnant woman on anything other than T4-only medications. Guidelines on using anything other than T4 medications in pregnancy aren't here yet either.

Whereas I do not feel confident that T3-only thyroid treatment is safe for pregnancy, I do feel that NDT and combination therapy of T4 and T3 can be safely used in pregnancy by a doctor who knows what they are doing. They will know if it is safe and the right thing to do for you. Testing levels every month, specifically the full thyroid panel, and adjusting dosage as needed, is key.

There is a consensus that the growing baby does not need T3 (active thyroid hormone), and that this is why T3 containing medications are unsuitable. However, whereas the baby may only need T4 from its mother's supply, the *mother* needs T3 herself to feel well. Many people cannot function without T3-containing thyroid medication (like me) and are unwilling to take T4-only medications because of this. If we don't feel well, we can't function, we can't work and our mental health suffers.

Although T4-only medication, such as Synthroid and Levothyroxine, is the most common thyroid medication taken in pregnancy, there are many women around the world who have had successful pregnancies and healthy babies on other thyroid medications, me included.

I had two healthy babies on NDT, one on Armour Thyroid alone and one on Armour Thyroid and Levothyroxine. You may need to find a specialist practitioner who will happily prescribe you a different option to T4-only synthetics if that's what you wish to explore. However, be aware that many doctors wish to move anyone not on T4-only medication to T4-only medication when they fall pregnant. As I explain in Chapter 7, this was the case with me.

However, I had no interest in changing medications because I knew what I felt best on, I knew NDT would be the best for myself and my baby and I also had no interest in destabilising my pregnancy by changing thyroid medication type during pregnancy. The private GP who prescribes me this thyroid medication also agreed with all those points.

I was closely monitored, with the full thyroid panel (TSH, Free T3 and Free T4) checked every 4 weeks throughout pregnancy, to ensure the dosage of my medication was correct. I was absolutely fine.

Why am I talking about this in the fertility section? Because once you are pregnant, it is not advised to change your thyroid medication type. So, if your body requires a different type, make the change *now* before you fall pregnant and have your levels and dose stabilised while working on optimising your fertility. Once you are pregnant, it is very likely too late to change or trial a change in thyroid medication.

A note for those on self-sourced thyroid medications such as NDT and T3, as I used to be one of them. Wherever possible, it is recommended to be on prescribed medication only when pregnant and this was one of my biggest priorities prior to falling pregnant - to move from self-sourced Thai

NDT to prescribed NDT. It is so much safer for both mother and baby during pregnancy if you're 100% sure what is in your medication, that it is consistent, regulated and safe, and that you have a doctor confident in dosing it. It is not recommended, for obvious reasons, to self-source and self-manage thyroid medication, but even more so during pregnancy.

Ensure You Are Taking Your Thyroid Medication Correctly

To get the most out of our medication, we should:

- Always take it at least 1 hour away from food, drink (excluding a couple sips of water), other medications, supplements, tea and coffee.
- Always take it at least 4 hours away from supplements (including prenatals) and medications containing Calcium (including antacids), oestrogen, Magnesium, Iron and antibiotics.
- Take it at the same time every day.
- Never skip doses.
- Ensure it is in-date and not expired.
- Always store it correctly (check the leaflet).
- If you've been prescribed a specific brand or type of thyroid medication which is working for you, then make sure that you're always given the same one, as some thyroid patients are given a generic substitute in place of their usual brand and end up feeling unwell again.
- A recent study showed that swallowing your thyroid medication with just one to two sips of water improved

thyroid medication absorption and stability for 100% of the participants.[16]

Ensure You Are Preparing for Thyroid Blood Tests Correctly

To ensure we are on the correct dose of thyroid medication:

- Take your thyroid medication *after* the blood draw.[17] [18]
- Stop any biotin supplement at least 48-hours before a blood draw.
- Test as early in the morning as possible, fasted.[19]
- Aim for your blood tests to be conducted at the same time of day each time.
- Reschedule your test if you're unwell.

Following these creates consistency when reviewing your test results and comparing them over time.

Optimal Thyroid Levels Table

Test Name	Example Reference Range	Optimal Range
Thyroid Stimulating Hormone (TSH)	0.5 – 4.4 mu/L	0.5 – 2.5 mu/L
Free T4	10 – 20 pmol/L	15 – 17.5 pmol/L
Free T3	3.5 – 6.5 pmol/L	Around 5.75 pmol/L
TPOAB	Less than 34 IU/mL	Less than 34 IU/mL
TGAB	Less than 10 IU/mL	Less than 10 IU/mL

Step 2: Reduce Thyroid Antibody Levels

Although many of you reading this won't know if you have it, 90% of us with hypothyroidism also have Hashimoto's Thyroiditis.[20]

Hashimoto's Thyroiditis is the autoimmune disease that causes hypothyroidism in most cases, and managing the Hashimoto's side of things can be just as important as correcting the hypothyroidism.

Why is it important to know whether we have Hashimoto's? Having Hashimoto's is a separate health condition to hypothyroidism and we all have a right to know whether we have an autoimmune disease. What's more, we *should* know if we have an autoimmune disease when going into pregnancy or starting a fertility journey. It can bring complications. For example, having one autoimmune disease increases the chances of developing another, and pregnancy is also considered higher risk in someone with an autoimmune condition.

Having Hashimoto's can also indicate that you have other areas of your health in need of support. Taking thyroid medication to address hypothyroidism is one area. Although conventional medicine does not have a treatment plan for Hashimoto's, more progressive / lifestyle medicine *does*.

When we talk about treating Hashimoto's, we refer to it as 'putting it into remission'. The word 'remission' refers to a reduction of the severity of a disease.

When it comes to Hashimoto's, remission is characterised by:

- Thyroid antibodies TPOAB and TGAB (Thyroid Peroxidase and Thyroglobulin) either being at zero or

within normal ranges. This typically means that Hashimoto's is more well-controlled and managed, as the attack and destruction of the thyroid gland is either halted or slowed down.
- No ongoing symptoms of fatigue, brain fog, muscle pains etc.
- Much less frequent thyroid flares / never having them anymore or hardly having any at all.
- Hypothyroidism may therefore be more stable and easily managed, too.
- Essentially, the progression of the disease is halted or slowed down.
- The Hashimoto's is not 'cured'. This is an important point.

Managing thyroid antibodies in pregnancy can be of importance, since experts state that thyroid antibodies cross the human placenta and could attack the baby's thyroid gland. Research has also shown that high levels of Thyroid Peroxidase Antibodies in particular can increase the risk of premature births. So, keeping Hashimoto's well-controlled for a healthy fertility journey and pregnancy can be helpful.[21]

The quieter your immune system response pre-pregnancy, the more likely that your immune system will allow successful embryo implantation into the uterine wall without risk for premature miscarriage (because of the overactive immune system attacking and killing off the embryo).

How do we reduce thyroid antibody levels?

Frustratingly, there is no one-size-fits-all approach to thyroid disease, whether that's hyperthyroidism, hypothyroidism or

Hashimoto's. When it comes to Hashimoto's, we see patterns of *what* reduces symptoms and antibody levels in a lot of patients and we can by all means learn from this, but there isn't one solution for everyone.

Common interventions that we see lower thyroid antibody levels include:

1. Going Gluten-Free (and Considering Other Foods)

One theory we see a lot is that gluten triggers the same autoimmune reactions that cause you to have Hashimoto's in the first place (called 'molecular mimicry'), increasing inflammation, which can mean worse or extra symptoms.

However, this theory is yet to be conclusively proven, so although I'm not saying it is 100% untrue, I am also not saying that it's definitely 100% true either. We don't know enough yet but we do have a lot of anecdotal evidence within the patient community and reported by thyroid experts to say that a lot of patients with thyroid disease feel much better when gluten-free.

Other possible reasons that thyroid patients feel better on a gluten-free diet and see lowered antibody levels include:

- that eating naturally gluten-free usually means a reduction in processed, high sugar foods overall.
- that a gluten sensitivity can lead to poor gut health, which can be indicated by a low absorption rate of minerals and vitamins. For example, low levels of B12, D, Iron etc.

If you are interested in giving a gluten-free diet a try to see if it helps, you may try eliminating it from your diet for three to four months and keeping a log of how you feel. You can also retest your thyroid antibodies to see if they come down.

However, there are huge benefits in screening for coeliac disease, an autoimmune response to gluten, before removing gluten. For example, diagnostic tests for coeliac disease require you to be on a gluten-containing diet so that the test can detect any antibodies to gluten. If you are already on a gluten-free diet when tested for coeliac disease, you will need to reintroduce gluten for several weeks before the blood test, in order to get accurate results. Having a formal diagnosis of coeliac disease, if you have it, is also important.

If coeliac disease is confirmed, then as well as a lifelong, strict gluten-free diet, a long-term treatment plan will also need creating by your doctor and dietician to ensure you're still getting the right nutrients from other foods. Monitoring of any intestinal damage and healing, as well as nutrient deficiencies is also recommended.

In addition to gluten sensitivity, you may also be sensitive to other proteins including grains such as rice, quinoa, and corn, driving thyroid antibody levels. Some people with Hashimoto's also react to dairy, soy, nightshades and eggs.

You may wish to trial going completely free of any possible offending foods for a few weeks to check if you do indeed have a sensitivity to them. See if you notice any difference in how you feel, or an increase in any symptoms after consuming them. It could be hours or a day later, but does it make you feel extra tired or give you acid reflux? You can keep a food diary and try an Elimination Provocation Diet (EPD).

The idea of the EPD is to initially remove all and any foods which may be making your thyroid health worse, before adding them back in one by one and looking for noticeable responses to these foods. Those wanting to try the EPD are generally advised to remove all potentially inflammatory foods from their diet for 3 weeks, which include:

- Gluten
- Dairy
- Corn
- Eggs
- Nightshades
- Nuts
- Legumes
- Shellfish
- Citrus
- Soy

After 3 weeks, the reintroduction of each food type can slowly begin. On a 'reintroduction day' you would choose one food type to reintroduce to your diet, eating around five servings in one day whilst monitoring symptoms over the next few days to determine if it needs to stay out of your diet for good.

Symptoms of a food sensitivity may include increased thyroid antibody levels, fatigue, heartburn, indigestion, bloating, gas, muscle aches and pains, joint pain, skin issues, brain fog etc. but can be individual to you. Foods can then continue to be added one at a time every few days and further signs for issues with these foods are recorded.

A lot of people will find they feel no different, others will have pinpointed one or two foods that are an issue and a small number will find that more than this are causing them issues right now. I only have an issue with gluten, for example.

Avoiding the other foods did nothing for me, so I gradually added them back in. Even for those who find they react to a few different foods; they may not need to avoid them forever. We don't want to unnecessarily avoid lots of food groups.

When it comes to goitrogenic foods, the general consensus is to eat them in moderation and that it seems they're only goitrogenic in their raw state. Therefore, many suggest that cooking them removes the goitrogens, or at least a large majority of them. Whilst consuming fermented and cooked cruciferous vegetables is preferred, occasionally eating small amounts of them raw should not aggravate thyroid conditions, so please do enjoy them! Eating a wide variety of plants is so important for your health. Goitrogenic foods include brussels sprouts, cabbage, broccoli, cauliflower, kale, radishes, peaches, pears, spinach, sweet potatoes, strawberries, soy, tofu, turnips and some nuts.

Overall, eating a nutrient dense diet is always going to be beneficial to thyroid patients in terms of supporting energy levels, optimum health, fertility and beyond. Foods that contain Zinc and Selenium in particular can be useful, since they provide nutrients that support thyroid function.

Sources of Selenium include:
- Meat – Chicken, Pork, Turkey, Beef
- Fish and shellfish
- Eggs
- Brazil nuts

Sources of Zinc include:
- Oysters, Crab, lobster
- Dairy
- Nuts
- Beans

You may have also heard about consuming enough Iodine. While it's true that we need enough Iodine to support thyroid function, excessive amounts can also be an issue. With iodised salt being readily available in most countries, most people will be getting enough from their diet as it is. If you consume a lot of seaweed for example, you could actually be taking in too much. A small intake of Iodine at 150-220 mcg a day is usually safe and potentially helpful.

The Omega-3 fatty acids found in fish such as wild salmon, trout, tuna, or sardines make these an excellent part of any hypothyroid patient's diet too. Hypothyroidism can increase the risk for heart disease as a result of higher levels of LDL, the 'bad' cholesterol, so fish rich in Omega-3 can lower the risk of heart disease. Fish can also be a good source of Selenium, as mentioned above.

Like Omega-3, other healthy fats such as olive oil, butter and coconut oil help to keep cholesterol at healthy levels, in order to produce the hormones our bodies need. Coconut oil also reduces inflammation, raises body temperature and gives the body immediate, usable energy. These should be consumed in moderation, however.

As well as their Zinc content, beans also contain a lot of protein, thus can be a great source of sustained energy, which, if you live with hypothyroidism, you may be lacking. They're also high in fibre, which can be helpful if you suffer from constipation, a common symptom of hypothyroidism too. You can use them in stews, curries and salads.

Fermented foods such as yogurt and kefir help to continuously stock your gut with beneficial bacteria, resulting in a stronger immune system and overall better health.

Cinnamon, ginger, garlic, peppermint, chamomile and turmeric are anti inflammatories, which may help to control your thyroid condition and promote better health. Let's focus less so on taking lots of things out of our diet, and more so on adding lots of variety in.

2. Consider Alcohol and Coffee

Keeping caffeine consumption low may also help with management of Hashimoto's, too. Caffeine can negatively impact your blood sugar. Blood sugar spikes cause cortisol to shoot up, which can tire out the adrenals and exacerbate hypoglycaemia, Hashimoto's and adrenal dysfunction. Caffeine may also irritate the gut lining and encourage acid reflux, headaches, migraines, poor sleep, poor thyroid hormone conversion and something referred to as 'oestrogen dominance'.

We are often advised to avoid consuming alcohol in pregnancy but did you know that it's also beneficial to avoid alcohol before you're even pregnant? I found that removing alcohol from my diet was the biggest factor that dramatically improved my thyroid health. Flare days hugely reduced and my thyroid antibodies came down a lot.

Alcohol can also contribute to adrenal dysfunction and deplete minerals and vitamins such as Magnesium, Zinc, Folic Acid, B Vitamins and Selenium, which are all important for fertility.

Which dietary changes did I make to optimise my fertility? I was already gluten-free, I gave up alcohol, kept caffeine low and then ate fairly balanced around that. I didn't give up sugar but I was mindful of not consuming too much of it. As someone who personally has a history of disordered eating, I am aware that information around diet can be triggering if you've previously / are currently restricting foods. Do know that I will never suggest that any of us HAVE to cut out ANY food types, so I present this information for each of us to make that decision ourselves if we still have ongoing thyroid symptoms or struggles to manage the condition.

Figure out what better controls your thyroid condition, brings down thyroid antibodies (if present) and supports your health and fertility.

3. Improving Gut Health

Hippocrates said: "All disease begins in the gut."

Your gut is home to your immune system, so when you heal and balance your gut function, it can improve your immune function too. Stress and an imbalance of gut flora can lead to poor gut health. I have experience with Candida (yeast overgrowth). Addressing this played a big part in getting my health back from Hashimoto's. More about this further on.

4. Supplements

As having Hashimoto's means having possible damage to your gut lining, stressed-out adrenals and more, low levels of key vitamins and minerals can occur. Because of this, there are some that you may wish to supplement. These include B12, Vitamin D3 (always take this with Vitamin K2), Selenium, Vitamin C, Iron etc.

Probiotics and Prebiotics are often recommended to help maintain a healthy gut, as are Magnesium and Zinc.

Supplementing Selenium has been shown to help lower thyroid antibodies, as has Vitamin D.[22] [23]

However, checking which supplements you need before starting any is really important and always check that new supplements will not interfere with your current medications. Run them by your doctor and only take what your body needs. More on this later.

5. Considering Infections

When treating Hashimoto's, it is also worth checking for infections anywhere in the body from the mouth to the gut and treating them appropriately. From mouth ulcers to tooth infections and H-Pylori, they can all affect gut health and drive thyroid antibodies.

6. Optimising Thyroid Hormones

Make sure you're on the right thyroid medication for you, and that your levels are optimal. This doesn't mean simply falling 'in range', but being in the place within the range, that you feel best.

To get your levels right, you may need to switch medication type (with the guidance of a doctor). A lot of patients have low Free T3 levels when on T4-only medication like Levothyroxine or Synthroid, as they fail to convert it to active T3. So, they may do better when adding in T3 to their T4, switching to T3 altogether, or switching to natural desiccated thyroid. It's about finding what works best for you. We're all different.

7. Supporting Your Adrenal Health

Having high or low cortisol can wreak havoc and contribute to Hashimoto's going crazy, too. You can do a 24-hour saliva cortisol test, testing four key points throughout the day, to test your adrenal function. We address adrenal dysfunction by improving sleep habits, exercise habits, diet and other lifestyle factors, including everything that contributes to stress. Stress is a major driver in chronic illnesses and autoimmune disease. Adrenal dysfunction is covered in detail further on.

8. Stabilising Blood Sugar

Blood sugar issues are common in those with Hashimoto's and can contribute to high thyroid antibodies. Again, this is covered in more detail later.

9. Low Dose Naltrexone (LDN)

Due to Hashimoto's being an autoimmune disease, LDN can be beneficial for those with Hashimoto's by reducing high antibodies, stopping the progression of the autoimmune disease or even reversing the disease. Besides improving endorphin production, LDN can also help reduce inflammation and encourage healing. This may be prescribed by your doctor before trying to conceive but is not necessarily recommended when trying to conceive or are pregnant.

Step 3: Regulate and Understand Your Cycles

Each month, your body goes through a cycle of hormonal changes. This whole process goes back to before you were even born, where you had all the eggs you would ever have already - around one to two million of them! However, only around three-hundred or so are released throughout your reproductive years.

Women are said to be most fertile in their twenties, with the general consensus being that around the ages of 19 to 27 we have the best odds, with a 50% conception rate per cycle. This decreases to 40% for those in their later twenties to mid-thirties and around 30% for those older than this. Rates for miscarriage have a similar pattern, at around a 10% chance for women in their twenties, 15-20% chance for those in their thirties, 34% chance for those in their forties and more than 50% when you reach your mid-forties.

Perimenopause

We're all familiar with the menopause, when your menstrual bleeds (periods) end around the age of 50, but less of us are as familiar with the perimenopause. The perimenopause can begin around ten years before the menopause and is characterised by your sex hormones (oestrogen, progesterone, testosterone) fluctuating before an eventual and inevitable decline; menopause.

When you are going through the perimenopause, your fertility may well be affected. The perimenopause may begin for some women in their 30's, however, it most often starts in your 40's.

What is The Reproductive Cycle?

Day one of your period is day one of your cycle. Yes, that's right - a new cycle starts with the arrival of your period. The first part of your cycle is called the follicular phase and usually lasts around 14 days or for half of your reproductive cycle.

During the follicular phase, the pituitary gland releases FSH (follicle stimulating hormone) which causes some of the eggs in your ovaries to mature and prepare for possible conception. FSH also creates follicles surrounding the eggs, one of which, around day 10, matures and grows. If more than one does this, it can result in multiple babies.

Oestrogen is produced (peaking around Day 13 along with FSH), causing your uterine lining to thicken and prepare for a fertilised egg, as well as luteinising hormone (LH) peaking, which signals ovulation. Your cervical mucus usually changes at this time, becoming more like 'egg white' to make it more hospitable for sperm. During ovulation, around Day 14, the mature egg moves along the fallopian tube. Some women, including myself, feel a twinge in the abdomen at ovulation, called 'mittelschmerz', and it may also be accompanied with spotting. The follicular phase ends here, and the second part of the cycle, the luteal phase, begins. During this phase, progesterone increases and you go from an oestrogen dominant first half of your cycle to a progesterone dominant second half. This increase in progesterone leads to the uterine lining (endometrium) thickening in preparation for a fertilised egg to implant.

After ovulation has taken place, there are two possible outcomes:

1. The egg is fertilised and implants in the uterine lining, starting a pregnancy.
2. The egg is not fertilised and around 10 days after ovulation (around Day 24 of your cycle) progesterone and oestrogen decline and signal for the uterine lining to shed and thus begins your period a few days later and you're back to Day 1 of your cycle.

All women experience one or two cycles a year where they do not ovulate, known as anovulatory cycles. This is quite normal, but if it is happening frequently, then considerations for thyroid issues, adrenal dysfunction, PCOS, anorexia, disordered eating, over-exercising etc. should be made.

Despite being led to believe for most of our lives that it's very easy to fall pregnant, many women find that when it comes to actually trying, it's not so. As you can see, a lot needs to line up perfectly for pregnancy to happen, including unprotected sex at the right time in the cycle, since you are only fertile in the few days leading up to ovulation and on the day of ovulation itself. Cervical fluid also needs to be the right consistency to facilitate sperm. Sperm mobility and good sperm health need to be in place for sperm to fertilise the egg and the egg quality needs to be good for it to successfully mature, implant and grow into an eventual baby. Miscarriages often occur due to an issue with implanting or missing chromosomes which affects how it develops. Whilst some of our fertility and pregnancy chances are in our hands, some are also not and this is important to recognise too.

When Cycles Don't Follow This Rhythm

In a study of 171 pre-menopausal women with hypothyroidism:[24]

- 77% had regular cycles
- 23% had irregular cycles
- 7% had heavy periods

Compared to a control group of women who did not have hypothyroidism:

- 92% had regular cycles
- 7% had irregular cycles and
- 1% had heavy periods

So, as we can see, women with hypothyroidism are more likely to have period complaints.

Heavy Periods

Undiagnosed hypothyroidism or less than optimal treatment for the condition is associated with a variety of menstrual issues. One of these is heavy periods, also called Menorrhagia. Heavy periods or Menorrhagia is defined as excessively heavy or prolonged menstrual bleeding, such as soaking through a sanitary pad every hour for several hours or more, passing large blood clots or your period lasting longer than five days, which is seen as the average duration of a period. Adenomyosis can also be behind very heavy periods.

Painful Periods

With heavy and long periods, you may also experience Dysmenorrhea, particularly painful periods. Some discomfort is expected when your body is shedding itself from the inside, but pain that leads to you taking time off work or school isn't something you should have to put up with. It commonly includes backache, headache (migraines) and stomach cramps (period pains). If yours are excessive or have you curled over in pain, they may well be caused by a thyroid problem, or other conditions such as fibroids, PCOS, adenomyosis or Endometriosis. Please have these evaluated by a doctor, as they can also impact fertility.

Irregular Periods

Irregular or sporadic bleeding, for example, going a month between menstrual bleeding, then two months before another and 3 weeks before another, can also be a symptom of hypothyroidism and is called Metrorrhagia or Intermenstrual Bleeding.

Amenorrhea can also come with hypothyroidism, which is when periods stop altogether. Amenorrhea can also be a sign of hyperthyroidism, so it's definitely worth having a full thyroid panel run to get a good insight into what's going on. With Amenorrhea, you are extremely unlikely to ovulate, which makes conceiving impossible. If you have irregular or sporadic periods this can be really frustrating and even anxiety-provoking. If your doctor will not run a full thyroid panel, you can order them yourself online from labs listed at the end of this book.

As well as a full thyroid panel, I would suggest looking into your salivary cortisol levels and checking for adrenal dysfunction (discussed further on in this chapter).

Short Cycles

Hypothyroidism and adrenal issues can also cause periods to come knocking more often than normal, a condition known as Polymenorrhea.

With this, you may find that your period comes more frequently than it should, every twenty-one days for example, instead of the average twenty-eight day cycle.

A sex hormone imbalance such as low progesterone and too much oestrogen, may be at fault, as a low progesterone level may mean that the luteal phase can't be sustained for long enough, so is cut short, bringing on your period sooner and harming chances of falling pregnant. The luteal phase is usually around 13-15 days long, so anything shorter than this can be an issue.

Hypothyroidism may cause a short luteal phase which can affect fertility. The luteal phase is the time between ovulation (the release of an egg) and the start of your period.

In order to become successfully pregnant, your body needs to be in its luteal phase for around fourteen days, to allow a fertilised egg enough time to successfully implant and start to develop. If your luteal phase is too short, a successfully fertilised egg may not have the chance to implant and so becomes removed from the body during your period. Thus, affecting the ability to fall pregnant.

Long Cycles

Oligomenorrhea refers to going 35 or more days between periods. Although associated more so with hyperthyroidism, it can still be present in hypothyroidism and Hashimoto's, too. This type of cycle can be a result of erratic ovulation, not ovulating at all or luteal phase defects.

If you have any of the period issues mentioned here, please have them thoroughly assessed by a specialist. They are often caused by thyroid issues, adrenal issues, fibroids, sex hormone imbalances, PCOS, endometriosis but also sometimes cancer. Do not ignore them.

Tracking your BBT

There can be multiple benefits to learning about your cycles and tracking your Basal Body Temperature (BBT). Your BBT is the temperature of your body at rest and your lowest temperature of the day. Thyroid hormones are important for maintaining a consistent BBT and if your thyroid hormone levels become too low, your BBT can drop. This may cause you to feel more tired and cold as a result. For menstruating women, a temperature between 36.1°C and 36.5°C is considered normal for the first half of their cycle, and between 36.5°C and 37.22°C in the second half. Lower than these and you may be under-medicated. Tracking your BBT for at least a month, though preferably for a few months, will help you pinpoint your own 'normal'. Some thyroid sources will say that a temperature between 36.5°C and 36.7°C is 'normal' and anything lower indicates hypothyroidism, but as you can see, if you menstruate then your temperature can differ wildly throughout the month, so this needs to be factored in also.

Tracking my BBT whilst working on resolving what my functional medicine practitioner referred to as 'oestrogen dominance' let me see the change in my hormones alongside physical symptoms also resolving (ongoing fatigue, migraines, cystic acne, irregular periods, gut issues and sleep issues). As these issues resolved and my irregular periods with no sign of ovulation gradually became more regular and ovulation became predictable, my BBT also reflected a more 'normal' or typical cycle.

Tracking my BBT meant that I became really in tune with my hormones and cycles which helped me understand my body so much better. I started to really get a hang of my fertile days and when ovulation was expected to happen. Using this information, I was able to optimise my fertility and know exactly when I was most fertile. It also helped me to recognise the signs my body gives when I'm ovulating or about to start my period, such as changes in cervical mucus, as well as changes to my BBT.

Here's How to Take Your BBT:

- Using a digital thermometer, take your temperature (usually under the tongue – follow your thermometer's instructions) as soon as you wake up and before getting out of bed. It needs to be your resting temperature, before you've had time to be awake for long or start moving.
- Record the temperature reading on a BBT chart when your thermometer indicates it has finished reading. These charts can easily be found online or with BBT tracking phone apps. I started off using paper charts but moved

to an app which was more convenient. I could plot my temperature each day and see it on a chart on my phone.
- A temperature between 36.11°C and 36.5°C is typical in the first half of your cycle (the follicular phase) and between 36.5°C and 37.22°C in the second half (the luteal phase). This can help indicate which part of your cycle you are in.
- A sudden temperature drop followed by a few days of higher readings (a "spike") typically indicates that ovulation has taken place. Ovulation usually happens around the middle of your cycle (e.g. Day 14 on a 28 day cycle). However, this can differ from person to person and conditions such as PCOS can impact when you ovulate too.
- The second half of your cycle (the luteal phase) should be at least 10-11 days long. If it isn't it may indicate that you are oestrogen dominant.

Charting your cycles and identifying when you are ovulating is a key part of optimising the chances of falling pregnant. Using a BBT thermometer, I would take my temperature as soon as I woke each morning, at the same time and before I sat up or got out of bed. A sharp drop in temperature followed by a sharp increase for three days showed when I was ovulating and when was the best time to try to conceive. After doing this for several months, I knew the pattern my body followed and knew that I ovulated around day 14 of my 28-29 day cycle.

Regarding ovulation tests, which detect a rise in luteinising hormone (which happens right before you ovulate), I found them to be very expensive to continue purchasing and it triggered anxiety in me when they never showed that I was ovulating (even when I was, as shown by

BBT). Purchasing a BBT thermometer just once was a lot cheaper. However, the benefit of an ovulation test is that it can tell you you're about to ovulate, whereas taking your BBT tells you when ovulation has already happened. You may wish to combine the two, it's up to you.

The 'fertile window' is generally defined as being the five days leading up to ovulation and the day of ovulation itself. This would be around days 10-14 of your cycle. Knowing when you're generally fertile by recording it for a few months (if not longer) before you attempt to fall pregnant, can make it easy to know when to have unprotected sex ahead of time.

Sperm can survive for up to five days inside the body, so having unprotected sex a few days before you even ovulate can still result in a pregnancy. Generally speaking, you want to ensure you are having sex, more than once if possible, during that fertile window (of around five days).

Other signs that you're at your most fertile time in your cycle include an increase in slippery cervical fluid (also called 'discharge'), as well as sore breasts.

If your periods are not very regular, are painful and you struggle to know when you're ovulating or are struggling to fall pregnant or maintain a pregnancy, then screening for other conditions such as endometriosis, adenomyosis and PCOS is recommended.

PCOS

PCOS (polycystic ovary syndrome) in particular is somewhat common with thyroid disease, and many of the signs and symptoms are the same too. On average, women with PCOS tend to have higher TSH levels and be subclinically (borderline) hypothyroid when compared to controls of the same age without PCOS.[25]

PCOS' irregular periods, non-ovulation, high levels of male hormones in the body (excess androgen) which can lead to excess facial and body hair, failure to conceive, weight gain, acne and hair loss from the scalp, can all be mistaken for symptoms of a thyroid condition such as Hashimoto's or hypothyroidism.

Hypothyroidism, and in particular, Hashimoto's, is more common in women with PCOS than in the general population. High levels of thyroid antibodies are found in one in three PCOS patients. [26]

If a person has either Hashimoto's or PCOS, the chance of being diagnosed with the other increases up to ten-fold.[27][28]

The cause of PCOS isn't well known just yet, but we do know that it often runs in families, just like hypothyroidism and Hashimoto's.

A diagnosis of PCOS is usually made following a ruling out of conditions with similar symptoms and a match of two to three of the following:

- Irregular periods which indicate that you do not regularly or predictably ovulate
- Blood tests showing high levels of male hormones, such as testosterone
- Scans confirming you have polycystic ovaries

Treatments for PCOS may improve your fertility and chances of falling pregnant. Clomifene may be used for those with PCOS and trying to conceive as it supports more regular ovulation. If this treatment does not work then another called

Metformin may be used instead. It works by lowering insulin and blood sugar levels in those with PCOS.

Endometriosis

Endometriosis is a condition where tissue similar to the lining of the uterus grows *outside* of the uterus, which can cause a lot of pain, heavy periods, and fertility issues. It can be really hard to diagnose. Medications and surgery may be performed to manage and treat endometriosis, however, if you're looking to have a child, you will want to ask if they will impact this. They can include, for example, using the contraceptive pill (birth control pill), an oophorectomy, a hysterectomy, removing some of the tissue or other surgeries.

Adenomyosis

Adenomyosis is a condition where the lining of the uterus grows into the muscle wall of the uterus, which can cause very heavy menstrual bleeding, pain, and even discomfort during sex for some. I was finally diagnosed with this after having spent my whole menstruating life with periods so heavy, I bled through the heaviest absorbency tampon and pad (worn together) every half an hour for the first couple of days of my period. My periods were so intense that I could not leave the house, would wear multiple layers of underwear in an attempt to contain leaks and missed school as a teenager. I was also chronically anaemic (Ferritin, stored Iron).

After checks for PCOS, endometriosis, fibroids and more were carried out, I was found to have Adenomyosis and started on Tranexamic Acid to treat this which has transformed my period every month. Not only can I leave the house, no longer require medication for painful cramps and not need multiple layers of underwear, but I can even swim on my period, something I never thought could be a possibility.

Assisted Reproduction

The use of fertility medicines, such as Clomifene, which helps increase the levels of FSH, as well as increases your chances of ovulation and number of follicles released, can be impacted by thyroid function and Hashimoto's. Artificial insemination and IVF (where the egg is fertilised outside the body and then transferred to the uterus) can also be impacted by thyroid health.

The demand for higher levels of thyroid hormone typically occurs earlier during the early stages of pregnancy when using these methods, possibly due to an additional strain on the thyroid gland. Therefore, closer monitoring of and optimising of your thyroid levels is crucial if you use these methods. Studies have shown that those with hypothyroidism may be less responsive to these treatments, however, more research is needed to ascertain why exactly. Other studies tell us that once transferred, fertilised eggs have similar success rates for survival in women with hypothyroidism and on treatment for this.

Step 4: Make a preconception plan

It is generally recommended that any woman wanting to fall pregnant has a 'preconception plan'. This is when you plan for your pregnancy several months before actually trying to fall pregnant, getting all your ducks in a row and your health optimised, ensuring you are in the best of health to begin your pregnancy.

After my miscarriage, it was recommended to me that I prepare my body for a minimum of six months before trying to fall pregnant again, as the egg released in each cycle generally takes this long to mature. The doctor told me that by doing this, it meant I optimised the quality of the egg being fertilised. You increase your chances of getting pregnant if both you and your partner are in good health and have taken steps to ensure this.

A preconception plan can include all the things listed in this chapter. Essentially, anything that is going to improve your health and quality of your eggs (and sperm in men) as well as making your body strong and healthy for pregnancy. I regret not strength training pre-pregnancy to get my body as strong as possible for pregnancy and birth. As a result, I am still working on resolving back pain caused by this.

Giving up alcohol, stopping smoking, eating a balanced and nutritious diet, reducing stress, optimising sleep etc. all help and will help a male's fertility too.

You can also assess your exercise routine and ensure you're getting plenty of movement as well as rest. Walking, running, swimming, yoga and strength training can all be hugely beneficial to our health and set our bodies up for a healthy pregnancy and postpartum period.

Some doctors will also recommend that you consider your weight and if weight loss may help you to fall pregnant during this period of preparing your body. While being a 'healthy' weight has been linked to better fertility and pregnancy outcomes, I would argue that embarking on a weight loss programme that sees you losing a lot of weight very quickly likely puts your body under more stress and can have the opposite impact on your health and fertility.

Looking to support or improve your overall health without focusing purely on the numbers on a scale or calories in food is often the best way to go about it. Weight isn't the only indicator of health. How much you exercise, what your diet is primarily made up of, your stress levels and quality of sleep and downtime is much more important. I chased weight loss for years and while I did end up in a much smaller body eventually, it came at the cost of a much worsened thyroid condition which was hard to get under control, crazy cystic acne, irregular periods, non-ovulation and poor gut health. My health was a mess. Dieting cost me my fertility as well as other parts of my health. When I changed my focus from weight to overall health and a reduction in thyroid flares and symptoms, my health transformed.

Yes, being overweight or obese can impact your fertility, but so can stress, cortisol and disordered eating behaviours, so I encourage you to consider the full picture and decide what promotes the best health picture in *you*. Often, when our bodies are happy and receiving everything they need, they shed extra weight with time and in a less stressful way.

I also want to talk about having a low weight or low BMI. If you are very underweight, then this has also been shown to impact fertility, especially if it also comes hand in hand with absent periods or irregular periods and other hormonal imbalances / impacts, or is a result of an eating disorder. Doctors may encourage you to gain weight to fall pregnant and yes, while this may help, you will also want to address if there are any reasons for a low weight, such as an eating disorder that requires support before you attempt to fall pregnant.

Just as many people in larger bodies can still be healthy, so can those in smaller bodies, but it's really not as simple as weight alone. It's the whole picture we want to be looking at; sleep, diet, exercise, stress management, how well any health conditions such as thyroid disease are managed etc.

Step 5: Look into 'Oestrogen Dominance'

Since the thyroid, pituitary and ovaries are all part of the endocrine system, it's not difficult to see why having a problem with one of these, may also mean having issues with another.

About a year after being diagnosed with hypothyroidism and Hashimoto's, I was told by a functional medicine practitioner that sex hormone imbalances were very common with thyroid patients and especially those with adrenal dysfunction too.

After testing, I was diagnosed with 'low progesterone / oestrogen dominance', which I was told created symptoms such as irregular periods, migraines, acne, PMT and more. Having 'oestrogen dominance' was apparently the reason why I was not ovulating and therefore, not fertile. This was confirmed via further testing, taking my basal body temperature daily and my periods being irregular (and often too short to support getting pregnant). However, whether 'oestrogen dominance' is real, is still debated. And hotly debated at that.

Oestrogen is a hormone primarily produced by the ovaries and is responsible for the growth of the uterine lining during the first half of a woman's cycle. Day one of this cycle is the first day of a woman's period. Progesterone is produced by the ovaries as well and its primary role is to prepare the uterus for conception. Both these hormones are present throughout your whole cycle but in varying amounts depending on where in this cycle you are. Oestrogen dominates the first half and progesterone dominates the second half of your cycle.

'Oestrogen dominance' is defined as oestrogen levels being too high in comparison to progesterone. The ratio is not optimal. However, 'oestrogen dominance' is not a term widely recognised in mainstream medicine and is used in more lifestyle / functional / naturopathic health spaces. Mainstream or conventional medicine will often dispute that 'oestrogen dominance' is real.

However, many of us report symptoms such as period complaints, acne, PMS, migraines, low libido and fertility issues, with a high oestrogen test result, which then resolve when a further test result shows more 'normal' levels of oestrogen, perhaps following the implementation of certain protocols which are said to target this imbalance.

So, 'oestrogen dominance' can be worth considering, however, conclusive evidence that it really exists is missing. In terms of medical professionals, naturopathic doctors and functional medicine doctors are often preferred by thyroid patients trying to combat 'oestrogen dominance'. I worked with a functional medicine practitioner to address 'oestrogen dominance', which I found immensely helpful when it came to resolving symptoms of acne, irregular periods, nonovulation, fatigue and more.

However, I am still undecided whether the protocols she had me implement really addressed any 'oestrogen dominance', or if they supported my overall health and these symptoms eventually resolved (and always would have done) anyway. But what I do know is that the protocols *did* help me.

In terms of fertility, my cycles became regular and predictable once more and I was ovulating again. Hoorah!

These are the interventions my functional medicine practitioner had me do:

- Ensure that you're eating plenty of fibre and that your bowels are moving regularly. Bowel movements of at least once a day are ideal, so eat plenty of fibre-rich food (though not close to taking your thyroid medication as it can affect absorption). You can also try Magnesium citrate supplementation to get bowels moving more regularly.
- Drink plenty of water throughout the day.
- Explore gut health and digestive enzymes to get your digestive system working more efficiently.
- Look for BPA and BPS-free water bottles, storage containers and minimise exposure through cosmetics and other household products. Reduce use of plastics.
- Avoid using hormonal contraceptives, which inevitably upset the oestrogen-progesterone balance and even when you come off them, can take years to correct.
- Products such as DIM and broccoli sprout extract can also help to clear excess oestrogen. Broccoli sprout extract improved my bowel movements, acne and migraines associated with 'oestrogen dominance'.
- Avoid stress. Easier said than done, I know! But stress is linked to affecting various hormone levels.

What can be frustrating is that whilst conventional medicine recognises that increased oestrogen levels can lead to increased chances of fibroids and breast cancer for example, they don't typically look to address the issue directly, looking at the body and endocrine system as a whole.

Many functional medicine practitioners will diagnose and treat thyroid patients presenting with symptoms such as acne, migraines, period complaints, low sex drive and more, with 'oestrogen dominance', but the evidence is lacking on whether this is a real issue that requires treatment. Many thyroid patients do report feeling much better after implementing protocols that claim to address this sex hormone imbalance. A lot of the suggestions in that list above are harmless to try, either way.

Step 6: Consider Your Gut Health

Often referred to as 'leaky gut' but more accurately called Increased Intestinal Permeability, this can also be a factor in our overall health and wellbeing.

Increased intestinal permeability and Candida (a yeast overgrowth) may be very common in those with hypothyroidism and Hashimoto's, since poor gut health is often cited as needing to be in place in order to trigger a thyroid issue in the first place. Improving my gut health was one of the biggest things I did to improve my health before falling pregnant again. It was one of the 'ducks' I knew I had to get in line.

My functional medicine practitioner improved my gut health by:

- Having me take probiotics and digestive enzymes.
- Drinking bone broth.

- Increasing fibre and water intake substantially. Eating a rainbow of fruit and veggies! Your gut loves food diversity.
- Using apple cider vinegar for low stomach acid.
- Using Grapefruit Seed Extract to remove excess candida.
- Being on the candida diet for a few months.

By addressing my gut health, the oestrogen dominance seemed to resolve, along with the high cortisol adrenal dysfunction (explained below) and my Hashimoto's went into remission.

Step 7: Support Your Adrenals

Adrenal dysfunction (hypothalamic-pituitary axis dysfunction) also seems very common in those with thyroid issues. I completed a four-point saliva test to check for adrenal issues and discovered that my cortisol was high all day long, contributing to symptoms of fatigue, struggling to fall asleep (feeling tired but wired), anxiety, hitting a slump in the afternoon, hot flushes, a weakened immune system and infertility. It was apparently driving the 'oestrogen dominance' and thus, I was not ovulating.

The slope of cortisol, which we typically see at its highest first thing in the morning and gradually dropping down over the course of the day, can be disrupted when we are chronically stressed.

Chronic stress may alter this slope to:

- low cortisol all day
- high cortisol all day
- low cortisol in the morning and high cortisol at night

This is what we refer to as adrenal dysfunction.

"Adrenal fatigue" is a term we hear a lot in the thyroid community. This well-spoken of condition concerning the adrenal glands has been debunked by the mainstream medical world on many occasions. So, is it real or not?

I think the truth lies in the details. The adrenal glands are part of the endocrine system, just like the thyroid. The most popular concept we see of adrenal fatigue is that the adrenal glands, which sit atop the kidneys and are responsible for producing hormones in relation to stress, get so tired out from stress that they eventually stop producing enough (or any) hormones. One of which being cortisol. We are told that this is the cause of "adrenal fatigue".

However, I find this to be an oversimplification and it's actually quite a terrifying claim that scares many people who reach out to me, thinking they cannot stop or reverse "adrenal fatigue" easily.

What I think is more accurately described as "adrenal dysfunction", is the cortisol slope that can be disrupted in a few different ways, or the 'HPA Axis'. "Adrenal Fatigue" may also be referred to as hypothalamic-pituitary axis dysfunction, as this is more accurate.

Symptoms of Adrenal Dysfunction:

- Struggling to fall asleep at night, or waking up a few hours after you do
- Feeling extremely tired in the morning, despite a lot of sleep
- Experiencing a mid-afternoon 'slump'
- Feeling more emotional than usual
- Depression or anxiety

- Ongoing fatigue that affects your day to day life
- Feeling unable to tolerate stress
- Hot flashes or sweats
- Intensely craving salty or sugary food
- Dark circles under the eyes
- Dizziness
- Mental fog
- Weight gain
- Low libido
- Extreme tiredness after exercise
- Unable to fall asleep despite being tired
- Heart palpitations
- Feelings of hypoglycaemia (low blood sugar) though test results are normal
- Hair loss
- Irregular Menstrual Cycles

There are two recognised conditions in conventional medicine, in association with extreme dysfunctioning of the adrenal glands: Addison's, which is a long term condition where the adrenal glands do not produce enough cortisol, and Cushing's, which is the opposite – where the adrenals produce dangerously high levels of the hormone.

Adrenal dysfunction may not be well-recognised in the mainstream medical world at the moment, but it is recognised in the lifestyle medicine world. This includes naturopathic, functional and lifestyle medicine. It is strongly felt in these circles that adrenal dysfunction (that is: an alteration in this natural cortisol slope) can cause symptoms and issues, though the cortisol levels are not as extremely affected as to the extent of Cushing's or Addison's.

I addressed adrenal dysfunction and brought my cortisol levels back to normal by fixing my gut issues and sex hormone imbalances already mentioned, with a functional medicine practitioner. The functional medicine practitioner said that the adrenal dysfunction, gut health and 'oestrogen dominance' were really a three legged stool, all impacting and driving one another. So, all three had to be addressed to restore my health.

Since stress is the cause, the simple answer to calming our adrenal glands and seeing cortisol return back to that expected, healthy slope, is to find ways to decrease stress, but it's important to understand that stress can come in many forms.

I'm not just talking about a stressful job, deadlines, financial stress or parenting young children. It also includes not getting enough sleep or rest on a regular basis, blood sugar imbalances (often caused by a high sugar, high carb diet), over-exercising, yo-yo dieting or restricting calories, ongoing family arguments and having no downtime.

Lifestyle changes are usually made to address stress, but it's very much individual to each person, as we need to look at what our stressors are. Prioritising sleep and rest, time to wind down and do activities such as reading, crafting, walking, yoga, baths or essentially anything that lowers your stress levels and promotes those feel good chemicals and hormones, is key.

Some people may need to reassess their work situation, create and maintain boundaries with friends and family around commitments, arguments and expectations, for example. Some may even need to reduce time spent with certain people who contribute to stress levels, if not stop seeing these people completely.

Ensuring that low thyroid hormone levels are corrected so that they are optimised can be important, as well as investigating possible food sensitivities which may be contributing. Eating gluten and consuming caffeine and alcohol were factors in my adrenal dysfunction.

Some vitamin and herbal supplements may support these lifestyle changes, such as ashwagandha (which is also sometimes discouraged for those with Hashimoto's), Vitamin C and B complexes. You may wish to consult a practitioner who recognises adrenal dysfunction, such as a functional doctor or naturopathic doctor.

Stress management and improving my mental health (especially when it came to having bouts of anxiety and depression) were also important when resolving my adrenal stress. Mental or emotional stress can really wear the adrenal glands out and exacerbate things. I saw a therapist for six months in 2019 to work through a lot of my long-term mental health struggles and improve my mental health for the long term.

Learning how to manage stress levels better was really important if I was to get my thyroid and adrenal health under control. Learning to say 'No' sometimes and better prioritise my time and needs felt good. Less overworking and more time away from social media also helped me feel less stressed in day to day life.

I also stopped over-exercising and forcing my body to do gym workouts and cardio that were limiting its ability to heal and worsening the high cortisol levels. Everyone is different but you must listen to your own body, and for me, cardio was making me feel worse for a long time. Many of us are over-exercising or doing the wrong kind of exercise for our hypothyroid bodies, and in fact making things worse. I was pushing my body beyond its limits by forcing cardio it just did not get on with, exacerbating adrenal dysfunction.

I stopped the gym workouts and implemented lots of long walks, swimming, yoga and joyful dance classes instead. I went back to basics and then gradually increased what my body was able to do again. It felt great to be able to exercise without feeling awful afterwards and instead feel energised. To support my adrenals, I had to really analyse the areas of my life causing and contributing to all kinds of stress - physical, emotional and mental - and tackle each of those areas one by one.

Step 8: Optimise Nutrient Levels and Supplements

When we have a thyroid condition, it's not uncommon to have some low vitamin and mineral levels too, and so many are important for fertility.

It is worth checking these where possible and supplementing low levels:

- Iron / Ferritin
- Vitamin D
- Vitamin B12
- Folate

Others you may not be able to test but can be beneficial to supplement with include:

- Selenium
- Zinc
- Probiotic
- Vitamin C (for adrenal support)

However, always run them by your doctor first. I'm not your doctor!

A good quality prenatal, which includes Iron, Vitamin D, B12, Folate – Methylfolate specifically, which is important for thyroid patients - Zinc, 2000 EPA-DHA Omega-3 (more than this can be toxic) and 200 mcg of Selenium can be taken while preparing your body for pregnancy too. You may then find you need to top up additional ones dependent on your own needs. For example, testing showed I needed extra Iron. Just make sure you leave at least four hours between your thyroid medication and any supplements containing Iron, Magnesium and Calcium.

In terms of Folate, this is important because it plays a key role in tissue and cell formation as well as DNS production in the foetus. It helps to prevent birth defects and neural tube defects. Neural tube defects typically appear in a foetus around 4 weeks of age, which is when many of us find out we are pregnant (this is the time you miss your period). Due to this, it is recommended that we start taking this supplement before we even fall pregnant. Think of that preconception plan I talked about!

Taking methylated Folic Acid over regular Folic Acid means that if you're in the 50% of the population who has the genetic mutation MTHFR, then it will still do what it needs to do. Those with MTHFR struggle with the methylation process, so it's much safer to assume you may have this issue and take methylated Folic Acid over unmethylated. Start taking methylated Folic Acid months before you start trying to conceive.

Step 9: Optimise Your Diet

Alcohol

As previously mentioned, giving up alcohol can be helpful in the management of Hashimoto's. However, whether you have Hashimoto's or not, the benefits of giving up alcohol while trying to conceive or in your preconception plan stage cannot be ignored.

I personally decided to give up alcohol for a couple of reasons:

1. as part of my preconception plan, in order to ensure my eggs and body were not affected by what is a toxic substance

2. because although I enjoyed the social aspect of drinking alcohol, I was very aware of how it caused thyroid flares and an increase in symptoms afterwards.

I almost always felt unwell after drinking alcohol, including digestive issues, acid reflux, lethargy, muscle aches and pains, headaches, acne and brain fog.

I eventually decided to give up alcohol completely and really didn't miss it. I did enjoy much less flare ups in my thyroid conditions though, as well as knowing my body was healthier for it. Also, by the time I fell pregnant, it wasn't a big deal to have to give up alcohol as I was already doing it and was used to it.

Blood Sugar

In terms of other dietary support, I also focused on the food I was putting into my body. Basing meals and snacks around protein and healthy fats instead of sugar and carbs helped to keep my blood sugar balanced which is often an issue with thyroid patients.

Important note: Blood sugar is *supposed* to go up after you eat, though there can be a problem when it spikes up dramatically, crashes back down and this repeatedly happens throughout the day, which can leave you feeling *urgh*.

Symptoms of imbalanced blood sugar can include feeling 'hangry', headaches, feeling faint and dizzy, feeling hungry again soon after eating, feeling tired, grouchy and irritable.

Many of us with thyroid conditions have adrenal dysfunction and stressors like poor diet and bouncing blood sugar levels can contribute to this.

When your blood sugar levels drop below normal, your adrenal glands respond by secreting cortisol. This cortisol tells the liver to produce more glucose, which brings blood sugar levels back to normal. Doing this repeatedly can cause abnormal cortisol output and can suppress pituitary function, worsening adrenal health and more.

The glycaemic index is a measurement of how quickly we burn food, and simple carbohydrates such as refined white sugar, refined flour, white rice, white bread, potatoes and carrots all have a very quick burn rate. Because of this, when eaten, they can cause a spike in our blood sugar, followed by a crash soon after. This is where more protein-rich diets can be better for us. Fat and protein have a slower burn rate. They are absorbed more slowly and gradually and so do not raise blood sugar levels as quickly as carbs and sugar do. They also keep us fuller for longer. Assuming enough calories are eaten to feel full, a person will be hungry again around two to three hours after eating protein, and about four hours after eating fat.

When we talk about fat, we often feel that it's something that should be avoided, but we actually require an adequate amount of fat for proper bodily functions (including those of our hormones). It's a focus on eating the right type of fats that we should have. Healthy fats play a big role in our mental health and moods, brain function, energy levels, weight management and hormonal health.

I ensure I consume enough protein and fat in every meal and snack, in order to keep my blood sugar levels balanced and promote ongoing, stable energy levels. To reduce the spikes in my blood sugar so it wasn't as dramatic, my functional medicine practitioner recommended I eat at least one third protein and fats to two thirds vegetables and carbs. More protein than this is even better.

Good sources of protein can include: meats, cheese, eggs, nuts, seeds, yoghurt, beans and legumes. Good sources of fat include olive oil, sesame oil, avocado, olives, nuts, seeds, peanut butter, flaxseed, salmon, chia seeds, eggs and seed butter.

We can aim to eat every two to three hours to keep blood sugar levels balanced and adrenals functioning well. Going a long time without food, such as with fasting or skipping meals, can place extra stress on the adrenal glands. We want our bodies to feel safe so they can concentrate on trying to get pregnant. If our body feels stressed, it may struggle to do this.

Overcoming My Eating Disorder

I have previously spoken online about my issues with disordered eating and overcoming it was also relevant to helping me conceive and be in a healthy place both physically and mentally, too.

I finally stopped yo-yo dieting and calorie counting and instead focused on feeding myself nutritious, wholesome food in the year prior to falling pregnant with my first child. This was a huge shift in how I viewed my health and how I looked after myself. I didn't realise until I had given up the calorie counting and restrictive eating habits, just how much they were making my thyroid and endocrine health worse.

Dieting can make you more hypothyroid (lowering Free T3 levels), encourage blood sugar imbalances and worsen adrenal dysfunction. My obsession with yo-yo dieting, restricting calories and focusing on my weight over how I physically felt were in fact not only hindering my ability to get my thyroid conditions under control, but making them worse, which affected my fertility too. These behaviours were impacting my menstrual cycles in the way that they were unpredictable and I was not ovulating.

In 2018, I took some qualifications in diet and nutrition and made an effort to focus on feeding myself really nutritious, wholesome food again. In particular, I incorporated a lot of the recipes from thyroid cookbooks - listed at the end of this book.

Eating with balance is crucial. We can all enjoy something sweet from time to time whilst eating mainly 'healthy' on other days. A lot of dieticians and nutritionists now talk about the 80/20 rule, eating nutrient dense wholefoods for 80% of the time and processed foods making up 20% of your diet at most.

Your body should feel safe when you want it to fall pregnant and restricting food does not promote this.

Step 10: Get On Top of Your Sleep

This one was harder than it sounds! Especially having adrenal dysfunction, there was a time when my sleep was all over the place. I would struggle to get to sleep, or wake up often during the night, wide awake at 3am and unable to get back to sleep. My adrenals were stressed and I sure felt it.

Making it a priority to stick to a sleep routine and get at least seven hours of decent rest a night, was helpful in maximising my fertility health. We are all told to aim for 7-9 hours of sleep a night. I made sure that I was getting into bed by 10pm in order to support adrenal health. A lack of sufficient sleep is associated with risks of lowered fertility.

I began to limit electronic usage in the evenings, particularly 1-2 hours before bedtime and made sure to leave work at the office. I had a cut-off for social media in the evenings and instead focused on bathing and reading in the hour or two before bedtime. I made it my routine to be in bed for 10pm every night, in a completely dark room, and after a few weeks it became the norm and my body was used to falling asleep around this time. Of course, addressing the high cortisol adrenal dysfunction in the ways mentioned previously was also important to restore my sleep routine.

It's also important to look at your blood sugar and ensure that you're keeping it well-balanced. Waking up at 3am for example, can be a sign of blood sugar being imbalanced and this may be helped by having a protein focused snack before bed.

You can also try cutting caffeine off from 2pm, as it can still affect you hours later and contribute to you not being able to get to sleep. Identify a point in the day after which you will no longer consume caffeine, if you're not giving it up entirely of course.

Exercising during the day also promotes a good night's sleep, so even if you're struggling with thyroid fatigue at the moment, getting in a fifteen minute walk can really help. You don't need to go mad with exercise and in fact, doing too much and pushing your body further than is comfortable can worsen any adrenal issues.

Sleep apnoea in thyroid patients has been linked to hypothyroidism and Hashimoto's, as those with these conditions are more likely to develop sleep apnoea.

Hashimoto's can cause obstructive sleep apnoea, which occurs when the throat is swollen and inhibits breathing, such as with a goitre (enlarged thyroid gland). Managing Hashimoto's effectively, often by trying to lower thyroid antibody levels and keeping them low, can help to manage this type of inflammation and improve sleep apnoea.

A note on Melatonin supplements for sleep: Melatonin in supplement form is often suggested in online forums, as this hormone can be used short-term to improve sleep, However, it is prescription-only in the UK and is contraindicated for autoimmune conditions as it can stimulate the immune system. It is also not recommended in pregnancy.

Step 11: Learn About the Spoon Theory

The spoon theory is a metaphor those with a disability, chronic illness, health condition or autoimmune disease, may use to explain the reduced amount of energy available for activities of daily living and tasks. This can be in day to day living or just during flare ups. It's a very popular term in the chronic illness community.

The idea of the Spoon Theory, created by Christine Miserandino, is that many people with a disability, chronic illness, health condition and/or autoimmune disease, for example, must carefully plan their daily activities to use their 'spoons' (unit of energy) wisely. Whilst people with no ongoing health issues do not need to worry about running out of energy.

'Spoons' are a unit of measurement used to track how much energy a person has throughout the day. A 'Spoonie' is the person managing their 'spoons' (energy). If you imagine that each activity requires a certain number of spoons, which will only be replaced as the person rests, then it's easy to grasp that if you run out of spoons, you have no choice but to rest until your spoons are replenished. You can imagine having ten spoons each day, and tasks such as showering or bathing requiring two spoons, and walking for half an hour (for example, home from work) requiring six. Those with a thyroid condition may have to work out which activities they can afford to do each day, so as not to run out of spoons (energy) and be left exhausted.

As other people without a health issue do not feel the impact of spending 'spoons' for mundane tasks such as bathing and getting dressed, they may not realise the amount of energy used by those who do need to plan their energy usage just to get through the day. They do not tend to have a limited amount of energy, as most daily tasks could never get close to exhausting them, unlike those with hypothyroidism or Hashimoto's, for example.

Even those who have their thyroid condition well-treated, like me, tend to be more at risk of over-exhausting and expecting too much of themselves, compared to others.

It takes balance, patience and a lot of practice to learn how to use our energy efficiently and get the balance right. However, managing a thyroid condition effectively and supporting your overall health for fertility includes knowing how to avoid repeatedly doing too much or sending signals that your body should be stressed and worried. It all ties in together.

Step 12: Learn About Men's Fertility Too

If you are having a child with a partner, it is also important to consider their fertility too, after all, it takes sperm (not just an egg!) to create life.

It is advised by fertility clinics that men should also partake in a 'preconception plan' stage, optimising their health for at least six months before trying to conceive. This can include limiting or removing alcohol, stopping smoking, reducing stress levels and changing a sedentary lifestyle to an active one. Considering supplements, such as Vitamin D, Folate, Omega-3 and Zinc can also be beneficial, since all four of these can impact the health and quality of sperm and Vitamin D also impacts placenta development. A man's health is reflected in his sperm.

There is also emerging evidence that pre-eclampsia and morning sickness in pregnant women may be due to the sperm quality in that pregnancy. Also, DNA fragmentation in sperm is linked to an increased risk of developmental delays and miscarriage. Lifestyle and stress levels impact the quality of sperm and its epigenetic tags, which determine how genes are expressed in your child.

Conclusion

All of these 'Steps' took me around three years to fully address, from being diagnosed with a thyroid condition to finally having them ironed out and ready to try and conceive (the second time around) but everyone is different and will have their own journey. I was still working on many of them when I conceived the first time around and although I'll never know for sure, it's a possibility that not having them fully addressed before I tried to get pregnant that first time, could have contributed to my body not holding on to that pregnancy. This is why I made sure to address everything fully before trying to conceive again, which did seem to help optimise my chances of falling pregnant quickly and healthily the second and third time around.

I especially do not recommend trying to conceive unless you know your thyroid levels are optimal, and you have your ducks in a row first. Focusing on getting your thyroid health and overall health to as good a place as possible before trying to fall pregnant is often the most responsible way to go about it. Miscarriages or other complications really aren't pleasant and if you can do anything to avoid them, it's worth it. However, we really do not know the true reason for many miscarriages, and this ought to be remembered too. Only so much is in our control, but I wanted to take control where I could.

Having a functional medicine practitioner, NHS GP and private GP all guide me on the steps I mentioned in this chapter, also made a difference. Again, it's important to state that what each of us need or do not need can vary a lot, so what your 'steps' are may differ to mine, but I hope that by sharing my experiences, they may help you.

If, after trying to conceive for 12 months, you have had no luck, it is recommended to see a doctor for a fertility evaluation. Depending on your age, this may even be after 6 months of trying. Unfortunately, not everyone is able to get pregnant naturally, so if you've followed the information in this chapter and are still struggling after 12 months, then assistive reproductive technologies may be useful to you. This can include fertility drugs, IUI, IVF, donor eggs, egg and embryo freezing etc.

This chapter was a big one… phew! Still with me? While incorporating these, remember: your body is amazing and we're aiming for a positive fertility and pregnancy experience here, so try to focus on what you *can* control and less on what you can't.

End of Chapter Checklist:

- ☐ I have made or have started a preconception plan.
- ☐ I have optimised my thyroid levels (TSH, Free T3, Free T4), considering whether a medication change is needed to achieve this.
- ☐ I have confirmed whether I have Hashimoto's or not.
- ☐ I have lowered my thyroid antibody levels (or am working on this).

- ☐ I have checked key nutrient levels (Iron, Vitamin D, B12, Folate etc.).
- ☐ I have started a prenatal supplement which includes Methylfolate, Zinc, Iron, Vitamin D, 2000 EPA-DHA Omega-3 and Selenium.
- ☐ I have considered supplementing with B12, K2, Vitamin C, Probiotics and Prebiotics.
- ☐ I have stopped drinking alcohol.
- ☐ I am conscious of my caffeine intake.
- ☐ I am not smoking.
- ☐ I am eating a variety of wholesome foods.
- ☐ I am having at least one third protein and fats in my snacks and meals.
- ☐ I have explored PCOS, oestrogen dominance, endometriosis and other possible coexisting conditions.
- ☐ I am tracking my cycles and identifying when I am fertile.
- ☐ I am taking steps to improve / support my gut health.
- ☐ I am supporting my adrenal health by unwinding daily, exercising in a way that supports my health (not making it worse) and setting boundaries for my mental wellbeing.
- ☐ I have checked my current supplements and medications with my doctor.
- ☐ I am optimising my sleep.
- ☐ I am implementing the spoon theory and am avoiding overexertion.
- ☐ Considerations for sperm quality are being taken into account.

Part Two: Promoting a Healthy Pregnancy

Positive Affirmations for a Positive Thyroid Pregnancy

My body is strong.

My body is powerful.

I trust my body to grow and birth my baby.

I embrace the changes my body is going through.

I trust my body.

I will work through any challenges as they come.

My body is doing what it needs to grow and nurture a healthy baby.

I give my body days to rest when it is asking for rest.

I choose to enjoy my pregnancy, even on difficult days.

I am my own best advocate.

I chose my medical team and I trust their care.

I am on a journey, growing and developing through this pregnancy.

I trust my instincts.

I will hold my baby.

Chapter 4: Being a Pregnant Thyroid Patient

If you're reading this chapter, then I'll assume that either a) you're pregnant and wondering what to do now or b) you're just super keen and super organised and want to know as much as you can before it even happens. And yes, this was me before I fell pregnant too.

Well, wherever you are in this journey, this chapter will continue to reassure you of all you can do to advocate for yours and your baby's health during pregnancy.

Everything included in this chapter has been collated from tonnes of research, speaking with medical professionals in regards to thyroid disease and pregnancy and also from my own experiences of going through pregnancy as a thyroid patient. I hope my experiences help you and also remove the need for you to spend countless hours Googling!

I want to give another reminder that we are all unique and that our bodies can respond differently to being pregnant too, so our needs can be unique as well. However, these are the key areas.

Step 1: Confirm Your Pregnancy ASAP

I confirmed both of my pregnancies at 4 weeks gestation. This is when your period is usually due. Besides actively trying to conceive and therefore having an inkling that I may be pregnant, other signs I had were:

- Missing my usual pre-period symptoms (light cramping, migraine)

- Dizzy spells
- Night sweats
- Feeling very emotional

I took a home pregnancy test as soon as I suspected, both times. Regular dye pregnancy tests are just as accurate as the electronic ones that show you writing on a screen; however, many people prefer how the electronic tests clearly state 'Pregnant' or Not Pregnant'. They often show how many weeks along you are, too.

By confirming my pregnancies nice and early, I could book in to see my doctor as soon as possible, which was still a few days away, but meant that I could get the right attention and treatment quickly. You can start testing as early as you want to but waiting until you're at least ten days past ovulation is probably best (this is usually a few days before your period is due), as getting negative result after negative result can be quite disheartening. Most pregnancy tests are most reliable from the day your period is due. I found out I was pregnant about two to three days before my period was due each time and I had very faint positive results. This is where the line is there but is very faint and can be hard to see due to HCG, the pregnancy hormone, not yet being very high. I followed these up with the electronic tests which clearly stated 'Pregnant 3-4 weeks'.

Step 2: Tell Your Doctor Immediately

I made appointments to speak to both my private GP (who prescribes my thyroid medication) and NHS GP the same day of having a positive test result. Due to availability of appointments, I saw the private GP first, just a few days after the positive pregnancy test, followed by the NHS GP a few days after him.

Both were very happy regarding the news and had no issues with my current thyroid medication and pregnancy. I was, however, booked in immediately for a full thyroid panel test to make sure I was on the right dosage to sustain and support the pregnancies. You should have this too.

For my first pregnancy, the NHS GP made referrals for me to see an endocrinologist and obstetrician as well. You may also wish to ask about this. He didn't feel the need to do this for my second pregnancy since he was more comfortable with my thyroid medication by then, as I'd already had a positive pregnancy experience the last time around.

Once you have a positive pregnancy test, your doctor really should be one of the first people you call. As the foetus doesn't have its own thyroid gland until the end of the first trimester, making sure that your thyroid hormone levels are optimal in those first few weeks is critical. The foetus is relying on your supply of thyroid hormone during this time, making the demand greater.

I would also recommend obtaining as much of your thyroid medication as possible to build up enough of a supply to see you and your baby through the pregnancy. There are occasionally recalls or pauses on production of thyroid medication due to issues we cannot foresee. My doctor was happy to prescribe me nine months' worth of my thyroid medication to make sure I did not go without it for any stage of my pregnancy and it really calmed my anxieties around this. Just make sure that any prescriptions do not expire before you'll use them.

In the UK, pregnant women are entitled to a Maternity Exemption Certificate (which is actually a plastic card) which covers the cost of NHS prescriptions and dental care. A doctor or midwife can submit the application for you. It lasts until around 12 months after your due date. The expiry date is stated on the card/certificate.

Step 3: Be Monitored Closely

All doctors involved in my care agreed that I needed the full thyroid panel (thyroid function test) checking every 4 weeks throughout my pregnancies, in order to make any dosage adjustments as swiftly as possible. Note that I didn't just have TSH tested, but the full thyroid panel. This includes TSH, Free T3 and Free T4.

TSH alone does not give the full picture and complete view of what's going on with your thyroid health. We should also be aiming for optimal thyroid hormone levels during pregnancy. This is different to just being in range, as explained in Chapter 3. Ranges for thyroid test results tend to change during pregnancy too, so make sure your doctor is using updated ones.

The ranges used on my thyroid tests while pregnant were the following:

TSH

1st Trimester: 0.09 – 2.83 mu/L
2nd Trimester: 0.2 – 2.8 mu/L
3rd Trimester: 0.31 – 2.9 mu/L
(Non-pregnancy range for TSH is usually around 0.5 – 4.4 mu/L)

Free T4

1st Trimester: 10.5 – 18.3 pmol/L
2nd Trimester: 9.5 – 15. 7 pmol/L
3rd Trimester: 8.6 – 13.6 pmol/L
(Non-pregnancy range for Free T4 is usually around 10 -20 pmol/L)

Free T3

1st Trimester: 3.5 – 6.2 pmol/L
2nd Trimester: 3.4 – 5.8 pmol/L
3rd Trimester: 3.3 – 5.6 pmol/L
(Non-pregnancy range for Free T3 is usually around 3.5 -6.5 pmol/L)

HCG, the pregnancy hormone, stimulates the thyroid gland, often leading to a lower TSH compared to before pregnancy. This is why test ranges change for pregnant women.

Your doctor should be keen to keep your thyroid hormone levels within the adjusted pregnancy ranges, in order to look after both your own and your baby's health. *Your* pregnancy ranges may be slightly different to mine, so they are just an example, please ask for yours.

It is normal and in fact the case for most women, that an increase in their thyroid hormone replacement medication will be needed during pregnancy. Your body needs crucial thyroid hormone more than ever at this time.

Many thyroid patients are found to need a thyroid medication dosage increase as soon as they are pregnant, and it is common practice for doctors to increase T4-only medication dosage as soon as a pregnancy is confirmed.

However, for other types of thyroid medications, this may be different. For example, in my first pregnancy, I was on Armour Thyroid medication and didn't need a dosage increase at all until I was almost at the end of my pregnancy. During my second pregnancy, where I was on Armour Thyroid plus Levothyroxine, the Levothyroxine needed increasing a few times in the first few months. This is why it's so important that we have our levels monitored closely, and that treatment and management is individualised to each pregnancy.

After all, a small study from 1990 revealed that although pregnant women taking Levothyroxine needed an increase in dosage to maintain good thyroid hormone levels in pregnancy, women on NDT medications (such as Armour) did not need an increase.[29]

According to the *Endocrine Society's 2007 Clinical Guidelines for the Management of Thyroid Dysfunction during Pregnancy and Postpartum*, thyroid medication usually needs to be increased in dosage, by 4 to 6 week gestation and may well require a 30-50% increase in dosage.[30]

In the *Journal of Medical Screening*, researchers demonstrated that pregnant women with hypothyroidism had a second trimester miscarriage risk four times the risk of women who were not hypothyroid.[31]

So, keeping on top of thyroid levels should be of paramount importance.

If a pregnant woman is 'subclinical' or 'borderline' hypothyroid, her doctor may wish to start her on thyroid medication or increase it so that she's well within the range to reduce the risk of miscarriage. The risk of miscarriage is higher in women with subclinical hypothyroidism, compared to women with normal thyroid function.[32]

NICE Guidelines, last updated October 2024 at the time of writing this book, state that anyone pregnant or planning to fall pregnant and has subclinical hypothyroidism requires a referral to an endocrinologist. It also says:

"Check that the woman understands there is likely to be an increased demand for LT4 (Levothyroxine) treatment during pregnancy, and her dose of LT4 must be adjusted as early as possible in pregnancy to reduce the chance of obstetric and neonatal complications."

It also advises that *"the woman is to seek immediate medical advice if pregnancy is suspected or confirmed"* when subclinically hypothyroid.[33]

The most important thyroid level in pregnancy is your Free T4. During the first trimester, the foetus doesn't have a thyroid gland and the only thyroid hormone that crosses the placenta during development is T4. Therefore, whether using T4-only preparations, natural desiccated thyroid or another combination of T4 and T3 medications, it is important to aim for a Free T4 level in the middle to upper section of the reference range. Being on T3-only medication during pregnancy is not usually recommended because of this lack of T4 for the foetus.

Additionally, if you have Hashimoto's, it's a good idea to keep track of managing this too, since some experts state that thyroid antibodies can cross the human placenta and attack the baby's thyroid. Research has also shown that high levels of Thyroid Peroxidase Antibodies increase the risk of premature births, so keeping Hashimoto's well controlled via lowered thyroid antibodies can be important too, as covered in Chapter 3.[34]

It was my responsibility to remember to book in for my thyroid tests every 4 weeks and it is yours too. Put a reminder in your phone, on your calendar, whatever works, to remind you to book tests when they're needed.

Step 4: Prepare for Morning Sickness

In case I experienced morning sickness, I made some plans with my doctor about what I could do to ensure I still absorbed my thyroid medication. After all, having enough thyroid hormone in your body is crucial in sustaining a healthy pregnancy.

My doctor confirmed that I could take my thyroid medication sublingually (under the tongue) if needed, although it *is* disputed whether the medication is still absorbed in the same way. We have a small pair of salivary glands under the tongue, where your thyroid medication pill can be placed in order to be absorbed straight into the bloodstream, bypassing the stomach so that even if you are sick shortly afterwards, you won't bring any of it back up.

It is worth tracking when your morning sickness strikes in case there is a pattern. It may make more sense to take your thyroid medication at a time which is clear of the sickness and lets you absorb as much of it as possible. My "morning" sickness would strike at midnight, with me taking my thyroid medication in the morning, so luckily, it didn't interfere, but many people experience morning sickness in the morning. For those taking T4-only medications such as Levothyroxine and Synthroid, these can be taken in the evening, however, T3-containing medications can keep you awake at night, so are often not recommended for this. If you take your medication at any other time than first thing in the morning and before food, then try to take it at least two hours after eating and an hour before eating again, to allow it to be absorbed with as little interference as possible. For example, if you have lunch at 12pm and an afternoon snack at 4pm, taking it at 2pm could work. The key here is consistency. If you have to take it after eating as opposed to first thing in the morning and before breakfast, be consistent so that your thyroid levels are easier to monitor and manage. Some women with morning sickness wake up feeling incredibly nauseous and need to eat straight away to relieve symptoms. If this is the case, then again, wait at least two hours after eating before taking your thyroid medication and ensure you don't eat anything else for at least an hour after taking it.

It can also be worth asking your doctor if an injectable version (or any other version) of your thyroid medication is available, should you experience morning sickness, as well as asking if your doctor can provide medications for sickness and nausea (anti-sickness medication) which may help you to keep your thyroid medication down.

Always discuss any concerns regarding your thyroid medication in pregnancy with your primary care provider or pharmacist, including if you are concerned that you're not absorbing enough of your thyroid hormone replacement medication. They may have other suggestions for optimising absorption but should always be kept in the loop with any changes you make, including how and when you take your medications.

Step 5: Revisit Supplements and Medications

I was advised by my midwife to choose a good prenatal supplement that included Vitamin D, Vitamin K, Iron, Vitamin C, B Vitamins, Folic Acid, Zinc, Omega-3, Selenium and Iodine. In terms of Iodine, not all thyroid patients tolerate it well nor need it, so you may want to approach a supplement containing Iodine with caution. That being said, I was absolutely fine taking a prenatal from a well-known brand with Iodine in.

As well as taking the prenatal, I chose to supplement some specifics on top of this. They included Vitamin C (to support my adrenal glands and immune system), Vitamin D (because blood tests showed I needed more), Iron Bisglycinate (also due to blood tests showing I needed more than the small amount in the prenatal) and Magnesium, which was to reduce constipation and muscle aches. I also took a probiotic throughout both pregnancies, to support my gut health.

We are told to not consume cod liver oil or supplements containing vitamin A when pregnant, as too much vitamin A can harm the baby.

You may have different needs and considerations, but please do review any supplements you currently take for safety in pregnancy.

Please also note that Calcium (including antacids), Iron and Magnesium should be taken well away from the time you take your thyroid medication. Not doing so can affect how much of your thyroid medication you absorb. Many people find that the solution for this is to take your thyroid medication in the morning and supplements with dinner.

As well as supplements, you will also need to confirm if all and any medications you currently take are OK in pregnancy.

My thyroid medication was obviously deemed safe to take throughout pregnancy (and actually crucial) but the medication I occasionally took for migraines prior to pregnancy, Sumatriptan, was not deemed safe. So, I was advised to avoid taking this wherever possible.

Once pregnant, you will need to get into the habit of checking all medicines, including paracetamol, ibuprofen, cough medicines and cold and flu medicines. Unfortunately, many are not recommended for use in pregnancy.

If you have symptoms such as extra fatigue, muscle pains, poor mental health, itchy skin or honestly, anything else out of the ordinary, do run them by your doctor in case a low nutrient level could be the cause, or something more serious. On the topic of itchy skin, your stomach, breasts, hips, thighs and bottom are all likely to grow and stretch while pregnant, so start applying a rich moisturiser or oil to these areas in the first trimester, daily, to prepare your skin for this. There is no guaranteed way to prevent stretch marks in pregnancy (most of this is genetic) but you can reduce how itchy and sore it feels by preparing your skin early on.

Step 6: Know Which Foods to Avoid

The typical food and drink we are advised to avoid in pregnancy include:

- Unpasteurised milk
- Unpasteurised cheese and soft cheese
- Uncooked mould-ripened soft cheese
- Uncooked blue soft cheese

- Pate
- Raw egg (Lion stamped eggs in the UK are considered safe)[35]
- Unwashed Vegetables, fruit and salad
- Uncooked/partially cooked meat (deli meats)
- Liver products
- Cured/fermented meat
- Raw/undercooked fish and seafood
- Swordfish, shark, marlin
- Alcohol

However, as someone who finds that being gluten-free helps to keep my thyroid condition under control and thyroid antibodies low, it was also important that I stayed on track with being gluten-free too.

If you also have dietary restrictions that help to keep your thyroid condition stable, antibodies lowered, symptoms reduced etc. then you'll need to keep on top of this in pregnancy too. Some people report that their food sensitivities are lowered or disappear in pregnancy but approach with caution. I definitely still felt the effects when I was 'glutened'!

Caffeine

We are generally advised that consuming caffeine in pregnancy is safe up to around 200mg per day. Regularly drinking more than this can increase your risk of pregnancy complications, such as low birthweight, and miscarriage.

To make this easier to follow:

- There is around 100mg of caffeine in a cup of instant coffee
- There is around 150-300mg of caffeine in one cup of brewed coffee from a coffee shop (if you have a favourite local coffee shop, look up their caffeine content or ask them next time you go in!)
- There is around 75mg of caffeine in a cup of tea (regular or green)
- There is around 80mg of caffeine in a 250ml can of energy drink

Step 7: Consider Your Exercise Regimen

Before pregnancy, I took long walks daily, did two 1-hour aerobic dance classes per week and 1-2 salsa dance classes per week. By the time I was 18 weeks pregnant however, I found I couldn't safely keep up with the salsa dancing anymore, and the aerobic dancing had stopped long before that! My reduction in balance and stability made these feel unsafe, so I reassessed.

Generally, exercise that has a risk of falling, including horse riding, gymnastics, hockey and cycling, are not advised during pregnancy. Exercise that involves lying flat on your back for long periods of time is also not advised, especially from 16 weeks onwards, because of the extra weight on the main blood vessel that is important for blood being brought back to your heart.

Side note on the topic of this: It is also advised that pregnant women sleep on their back after 28 weeks of pregnancy, to reduce the risk of stillbirth. This is due to a reduced flow of oxygen and blood to the baby when you sleep on your back. If you wake up on your back, try not to panic, instead move back on to your side. A long pregnancy pillow can really help to keep you in a side sleeping position too.

I started an antenatal yoga class at 13 weeks, which was a great balance between movement and relaxation. I was stretching and moving, but it was gentle and adaptable and helped to reduce my stress levels.

As well as yoga, I kept up daily walks throughout pregnancy and also began swimming once a week when I stopped the salsa classes. Swimming felt amazing when my body was achy and heavy. Walking, swimming and yoga worked really well for me. I still got a good workout (especially from swimming) but didn't feel completely wiped out. The yoga moves I learned also came in handy later on in pregnancy when I had a lot of trapped wind! They can also be used in labour. I can't recommend pregnancy yoga enough.

If you enjoy strength training, this may be continued in pregnancy if you feel well enough.

During the first and third trimester especially, you can feel incredibly tired, so listen to your body and rest when it is needed. As a general rule, you'll know if you've got the intensity right as you should be able to hold a conversation when you exercise and are pregnant. If you feel out of breath, it may be too intense and a sign to slow things down. Please read Chapter 5 for more information on exercising in pregnancy!

Step 8: Pick Up Books

I read a lot of books to feel clued up about my pregnancy. This helped me feel reassured that I was doing as much as possible to look after both myself and the baby.

Books I found useful included:

- **The Positive Birth Book: The Guide to Pregnancy, Birth and the Early Weeks** by Milli Hill
- **The Pregnancy Encyclopedia** by DK
- **What to Expect When You're Expecting** by Heidi Murkoff
- **Healing Your Body Naturally After Childbirth** by Dr. Jolene Brighten

Find my full list of resources at the back of this book!

Step 9: Avoid Illness Where Possible

Vaccines are always a controversial topic, but yes, I did opt to have all of my pregnancy vaccines, including the flu and whooping cough, with no issues to report. When I contracted the flu at seventeen-years-old, I ended up in intensive care, on breathing support. Therefore, the flu vaccination is something I choose to have every winter. These decisions are always personal however, and only you know what you're comfortable doing and what is in the best interest of your health and your baby's health. There is also now the Covid-19 vaccine which is widely recommended to all those pregnant.

I was also more aware of catching other illnesses whilst pregnant, so I made sure to take all my supplements regularly to support my immune system and health, and I washed my hands frequently and took extra measures to avoid catching bugs or colds. I really didn't want to add sickness on top of pregnancy, hypothyroidism and Hashimoto's. Many of us with autoimmune hypothyroidism can be more susceptible to picking up illness and then take weeks to recover from them.

I wasn't ill often in my first pregnancy but I was ill a lot in my second, due to also having a toddler at the time who was bringing back a constant stream of germs from childcare. There is only so much you can do! Any time I was unwell in my second pregnancy, it hit me really hard, a lot harder than if my son and husband also got the illness. As I explain in Chapter 7, one sickness bug landed me in hospital for three days with preterm contractions from dehydration.

It is worth noting the effects on Hashimoto's during pregnancy. Due to changes in how the immune system works in pregnancy (in order to protect the baby and not reject it as a foreign, dangerous invader) the immune system 'quietens down', which is why pregnant women come down with coughs, colds and bugs easier, but also why many see their autoimmune diseases, like Hashimoto's, go into remission or otherwise calm down a lot, too.

Step 10: Schedule a Dentist Check-Up

I experienced jaw stiffness and pain in the first trimester of my first pregnancy, so I booked to see the dentist for a check-up. Thankfully, she didn't see anything that was a cause for concern. It later reemerged when my firstborn was six months old and we found out it was a wisdom tooth causing trouble. It's a good idea to have your dental health evaluated whilst pregnant. In the UK, you are entitled to free NHS dental treatment when you're pregnant (and for 12 months after your baby is born). See my note on the Maternity Exemption Certificate in Step 2 of this chapter.

Step 11: Rest During Thyroid Flares

Thyroid flares are quite a common part of having thyroid disease, and with the added stress of pregnancy, they can become more common at this time in your life too. Whilst I did expect some thyroid flare days when pregnant, I felt very lucky in that they were certainly not frequent. When they hit, I was mindful about looking after myself.

Symptoms of a thyroid flare include:

- Increased fatigue
- Heaviness (as if your body is being weighed down)
- Worsened mental health
- Brain fog
- Migraines
- Flu-like symptoms (aches and pains)
- Dizziness
- Switching between feeling really cold and really hot

A thyroid flare is defined by an increase in symptoms of your thyroid condition, usually due to one of the causes listed below. A flare usually lasts for somewhere between one day to a few weeks. The most common amount of time reported is a few days.

THE POSITIVE THYROID PREGNANCY BOOK

The most common causes of flares are:

- Drinking alcohol
- Eating a lot of sugary or processed food / not giving your body enough nutrient dense food. (for example, it may follow the Christmas period when a lot more processed food is consumed and replaces more nutrient-dense and a wider range of foods)
- Consuming a food your body does not like – an allergen, intolerance or sensitivity. (such as gluten or dairy)
- Mental or physical overexertion (may occur after a busy vacation / holiday, lots of social events or busy work period)
- High amounts of stress
- Not sticking to a predictable sleep routine
- Viral, bacterial, fungal infections (illnesses caught from family members, ear infections, tonsillitis etc.)
- Being on your period or due to start your period (hormonal fluctuations)
- Pregnancy (more hormonal fluctuations, plus it's easier to overexert yourself!)

So, as you can see, just being pregnant may trigger more of them for you.

Looking after yourself during thyroid flares is important, as you are looking after both yourself and your growing baby, needing to do what is best for the two of you. Most of the time, you will need to prioritise resting where you can and avoid being too hard on yourself.

Many people still need to work while pregnant, so taking frequent breaks, staying hydrated, eating well, wearing comfortable clothing, sitting down, keeping warm, relaxing in baths after work and limiting physical activity during a flare, all help. Choose nourishing food, consider bone broths and if you can't cook and must order takeaway, consider the many 'healthy takeaway' options now available. More nutrient-dense food that is going to help your body recover quicker, can really go a long way. I avoid sugar and caffeine on flare days, too.

On my flare days where I had to work or otherwise didn't have the luxury of resting in front of the TV, I compromised. I limited how much work or other commitments would impede my recovery from a flare. For example, I sought permission to work from home, working altered hours until the flare had passed, replacing walking to and from work with transport to save energy, or otherwise speaking to my line manager about suitable adjustments. If making changes surrounding my work wasn't an option, at the very least I supported recuperating outside of work as much as possible by limiting how much unnecessary activity I did and maximising resting and recuperation time instead. We have to say "no" sometimes.

During my second pregnancy, I was also looking after my two-year-old son, which made resting more difficult. On flare days where I still had to parent, I found that these helped me:

- Eat as nourishingly as you can. This is not always easy when you're ill and you have children screaming at you, but you can keep it simple. For example, when I am feeling well, I will cook a large bean chilli for dinner, putting a few portions in the freezer for *flare day me* to heat up in the oven.
- I'll stay home wherever I can, cancel social plans and anything nonessential. Yes, my child still requires looking after but a lot of errands can wait another day when I am hopefully more recuperated.

- I look for ways my child and I can do lower energy activities, for example: a movie day, PJ day, stickers and colouring books, sharing a bath if they're still small (it's not as relaxing as a bath on my own, but it still eases the aches and pains!), getting them in the garden to play while I sit with a blanket and hot drink on the doorstep and even playing in bed (hiding under covers).
- Use a hot water bottle. I'll carry it around with me as we play on the floor or move around. Just holding it helps me feel a little brighter as I'm often cold on flare days.
- I will always ensure that I go to bed early on a flare day. Once my little one is in bed, so am I! If they napped, I would nap too.
- Pull in Support. Not all of us are lucky enough to have friends and family close by. I have often struggled with feeling lonely and isolated on tough thyroid days. However, for those that *do* have someone who can help: Can they watch the kids for an hour while you rest in bed? Can they bring you a meal? Can your children have a playdate out the house? Perhaps you know one of their friend's parents quite well, who would welcome them coming round to play for an hour or two while you rest?

I chose to save up for a spa day during both pregnancies and took them around 30 weeks pregnant. I suspected that my body would need it by then and I was right!

Step 12: Confirm If You Are 'High Risk'

A 'high-risk pregnancy' is one of greater risk to the mother or her baby, compared to a more straightforward pregnancy.

Having hypothyroidism and/or Hashimoto's are considered to be risk factors.[36]

Several factors can make a pregnancy high risk, including existing health conditions and health issues that happen before or during pregnancy:

- Pre-existing health conditions, such as: high blood pressure, PCOS, diabetes, kidney disease, autoimmune diseases, thyroid issues
- Obesity
- Drug/alcohol/cigarette use
- Age: teenagers, older mothers-to-be (35+)
- Twin, triplet+ pregnancies
- Having had a previous preterm birth (born before 37 weeks of pregnancy)
- Birth defects or genetic conditions in the baby
- Health conditions which develop during pregnancy, such as: pre-eclampsia, gestational diabetes, Low Papp-A, Abnormal liver function

Both hypothyroidism and Hashimoto's are considered to be risk factors, however, whether you are personally considered as 'high risk' will be decided on an individual basis. After all, each pregnancy is different, including the mother-to-be and her personal health situation. What may be considered a risk to one pregnancy, may not be for another.

In my first pregnancy, the NHS GP referred me to both an obstetrician and endocrinologist as he initially considered me to be 'higher risk', though not for my hypothyroidism or Hashimoto's alone. The thyroid medication I was taking,

Armour Thyroid, was unfamiliar to him as well as much of the NHS.

After seeing both the endocrinologist and obstetrician, I was discharged from both and any label of 'possibly being high risk' was withdrawn.

My second pregnancy was classed as high risk due to non-thyroid related complications. The doctors were not concerned about my medication this time either, but I had another complication which put myself and the baby at higher risk for issues. (This is all covered in Chapter 7)

If you're experiencing complications of your thyroid condition during pregnancy, e.g. levels fluctuating quite a lot or experiencing blood pressure concerns, then you may be considered 'high risk'. If you are also on a privately prescribed or self-sourced thyroid medication, or considered to be 'borderline' hypothyroid and not on treatment, these may also play into whether you are 'high risk'.

It's also worth noting that if you're 'borderline' hypothyroid, your doctor may wish to start you on thyroid medication or increase it so that you're well within range to reduce risk of miscarriage. The risk of miscarriage is higher in women with subclinical hypothyroidism, compared to women with normal thyroid function (euthyroidism).[37]

Subclinical hypothyroidism in the mother is also associated with a higher risk of pre-eclampsia.[38]

Pre-eclampsia is a pregnancy complication that involves high blood pressure and protein found in urine. It can also cause damage to the liver and kidneys. Symptoms include high blood pressure, headaches, vision changes, abdominal pain, swelling of the feet, ankles, hands or face and nausea or sickness. With its link to thyroid levels, it's worth knowing the signs and symptoms.

Pregnant women with autoimmune hypothyroidism also have an increased risk of developing gestational diabetes. This is a condition I was monitored for closely as the midwives told me I was slightly more likely to develop it, but thankfully never did. Symptoms include increased thirst, frequent urination, fatigue, a dry mouth, vision changes, nausea or sickness.

Generally, it seems that women on standard T4 thyroid medication such as Levothyroxine or Synthroid and are well and easily managed, are not considered to be 'high risk', but your doctor or healthcare team may have individual concerns about your particular situation.

You can keep risks low by following the advice in this chapter, such as informing your doctor as soon as you are pregnant, having regular blood tests, stopping alcohol, stopping smoking and more.

Although women with thyroid issues are more likely to have obstetric complications than women without thyroid disease, it is important to know that most women with thyroid disease do not experience complications in pregnancy and in fact have a straightforward pregnancy and birth. Ensuring your thyroid levels are optimised is a key part of this.

Step 13: Raise All and Any Concerns

Whenever I had any concerns during pregnancy, I raised them with my healthcare team as soon as they cropped up. Heart palpitations, vaginal bleeding, skin itchiness, migraines with aura and sciatica… it was important to raise them all and get thoroughly checked out.

Occasionally, we had to take extra thyroid tests to ensure that my thyroid condition wasn't behind any of them. So please raise all concerns early on. As they say: Better safe than sorry.

Postnatal depression is a term many of us are familiar with, but antenatal depression, experienced when you are pregnant, is lesser known. I experienced antenatal depression during my second pregnancy, which was really hard. My thyroid hormone levels dropped suddenly and frequently until I was around five months pregnant, which no-doubt contributed to this diagnosis. Please keep in mind the role that your thyroid hormones play in mental health, should you be experiencing antenatal depression too, and please reach out for support. Upon speaking to my midwife about it, I realised it was a lot more common than I thought and she could point me towards further support.

Step 14: Plan Your Maternity / Paternity Leave

While you are pregnant, it is crucial to look ahead and plan for your maternity and paternity leave. Many factors will play into how much time you take off from work and what a return to work may look like, as well as the use of childcare. Confirm what options are available with your workplace and what works for you from a financial perspective, too.

When it comes to factoring in your thyroid health and wanting to keep on top of this so that you can enjoy parenthood as much as possible, looking for a good work-life balance helps. I chose to return to work for two days a week initially, increasing this to three days a week after a few months. We used childcare that staggered my workdays and solo parenting days, so that I could stagger my energy usage (my workdays involve sitting at a desk whereas my children *do not* sit still!). Some families like grouping work and childcare days together, for example, working Wednesday to Friday. Whereas a staggered Monday, Wednesday, Friday routine may work better for you and your health. It will depend on what type of work you do too.

My partner took off as much paternity leave as he could each time, adding annual leave days on to his statutory amount to extend this. I found that I hugely benefited from the extra support that this gave me in the early days of managing a new baby alongside my thyroid condition. We could tag in and out to allow each other to sleep or rest up, and he would also bring me nutritious snacks, meals and drinks while I was 'nap-trapped' or breastfeeding and unable to move! Having this support around, whether in the form of a partner, your parents (who may be able to stay with you for a while) or friends can make a huge difference to your health postpartum. Take some time to plan the first few months postpartum before the baby comes.

Also, if you can batch cook some bean chillis, bolognese, homemade curry sauces etc. and store them in the freezer while you're pregnant, you'll be so grateful for it when you have a newborn and need quick, nutritious meals.

Another decision you may wish to think about before your baby is born is whether you wish to breastfeed, formula feed or combi-feed. Breastfeeding helps nourish your baby's gut health early on, promotes bonding, is often easier to digest, and reduces the chances of them developing a whole range of health conditions such as asthma, eczema, ear infections, respiratory infections and SIDS (sudden infant death syndrome). However, breastfeeding is not always possible or easy for many reasons. I explore this further in Chapter 11.

Conclusion

Looking after your thyroid health during pregnancy is very important.

Associated risks of improperly managed thyroid conditions during pregnancy include abnormal or low thyroid hormone levels, which can unfortunately lead to complications or increases in risk of miscarriage, pre-eclampsia, anaemia, stillbirth and more.

Some researchers believe that one factor in the development of autism is severe hypothyroidism in the mother.[39]

However, the vast majority of pregnant women with thyroid conditions have very normal and uneventful pregnancies. Let's remember this important fact!

Having a functional medicine practitioner, NHS GP and private GP all involved in my care made a difference for me. At one point, an endocrinologist and an obstetrician were also involved. Chapter 6 covers different types of doctors you may wish to involve.

Predicting with complete certainty what a thyroid patient's health is going to be like during pregnancy and after giving birth is impossible, but it doesn't mean you can't be prepared. Whereas some women with thyroid issues report feeling worse when pregnant, for many others, they feel better.

You can prepare for needing more support than others by building a support network prior to the baby's arrival, such as people you can count on to help cook meals, do laundry or otherwise help you out. I also enjoyed researching local baby groups while pregnant, so I had an idea of support groups available to me on certain days too.

If you can prioritise being as prepared as possible, as well as that any birth partner or spouse is as involved as they can be (encourage them to read this book!), then it will really help when you go through the lifechanging event of becoming a parent.

Thyroid symptoms such as brain fog, fatigue and mood swings can increase during pregnancy, so it's useful if your support is present to ask questions and be an extra pair of ears to listen and remember key information at medical appointments or prenatal classes. It may be that the pregnant thyroid patient feels more easily overwhelmed during pregnancy, so be in this together. It will help you both.

The chances are that thyroid levels will go up and down throughout pregnancy and this may mean that swings between better health and worse health days can occur. Therefore, it will really help if a partner is involved.

A list of items that helped me with pregnancy symptoms:

- A bouncy pregnancy / exercise ball - for back pain, general exercising, use during labour and also for bouncing baby to sleep after birth!
- A yoga mat for pregnancy yoga.
- Non wired, non-padded, stretchy and comfy bralettes / bras.
- A pregnancy pillow - My back and pelvic pain were much better with this support.
- Hot water bottles for back and hip pain.
- Magnesium Citrate helped relieve constipation.

End of Chapter Checklist:

- ☐ I have had a positive pregnancy test to confirm my pregnancy and have been given an estimated due date.
- ☐ I have booked an appointment with my doctor/s to inform them and make a plan.
- ☐ I have asked if it is possible to 'stock up' on enough thyroid medication to last me through my pregnancy.
- ☐ In the UK: I have applied for a Maternity Exemption Certificate.
- ☐ I have agreed with my doctor how often my thyroid panel testing will be conducted (ideally every 4-6 weeks). And I have put reminders to book these / for when they are due in my calendar.
- ☐ I have confirmed that adjusted lab ranges for pregnancy will be used.
- ☐ I have asked my doctor if I require an immediate increase in my thyroid medication.
- ☐ Subclinical hypothyroidism only: I have asked to start medication.
- ☐ I have made a plan in preparation for possible 'morning sickness'.
- ☐ I have started a prenatal supplement and revisited whether my other supplements and medications are still safe / necessary for pregnancy.
- ☐ I am leaving enough time between taking my thyroid medication and any other medications or supplements.
- ☐ I am confident in which food and drinks I should be avoiding in pregnancy.
- ☐ I have reassessed my exercise and if it's still making me feel good. I have explored pregnancy yoga.

- ☐ I am checking out other books on pregnancy and postpartum (recommendations at the back of this book).
- ☐ I have considered whether I wish to breastfeed, formula feed, etc.
- ☐ I have considered my pregnancy vaccinations (flu, covid, whooping cough etc.)
- ☐ I have booked in for a general dentist check-up.
- ☐ I am resting during flares.
- ☐ I have asked if my pregnancy is high risk and what impacts this may have on my pregnancy and birth.
- ☐ I am raising all questions and concerns.
- ☐ I have made a plan for postpartum and maternity leave.
- ☐ My spouse / birth partner / family has also read this chapter!

Chapter 5: Exercising While Pregnant

Before pregnancy, I had enjoyed carving out an exercise routine I enjoyed and that supported my health as a thyroid patient. I took a walk every day, dance classes and other cardio classes weekly and occasionally played badminton. However, by the time I was approaching the third trimester of my first pregnancy, I found these classes exhausting and no longer safe, given my tendency to lose my balance with a nice, round bump! We're all different and may find that different types of exercise work for us, so this chapter will explore this.

If you haven't already, now is the time to invest in some new clothes to support your growing bump and body and allow you to exercise as comfortably as possible.

You will need:

- Bigger, stretchy underpants (a lot of women buy a size up in regular briefs)
- Non-wired maternity bras or bralettes (often being remeasured and refitted every few months throughout pregnancy)
- Maternity leggings and loose tops that accommodate a growing bump
- Comfy trainers - feet often change shape and size in pregnancy, so don't be surprised if you need to size up!
- A maternity swimming costume / swimsuit

How To Exercise Safely

Exercise is an important part of a healthy lifestyle and pregnancy, but it's important to get the balance right.

Know Your Limits

Exercising with thyroid disease and pregnancy may feel difficult and if you were a more active person pre-pregnancy, it can be hard to accept that your exercise regimen may need to change so as not to make yourself feel more unwell. After all, repeatedly over-exercising or pushing too far can lead to thyroid flares and setbacks in your health. Learning to get the balance right and relearning what your body is comfortable doing now that it is carrying and growing life, is important.

Repeatedly engaging in overly demanding exercise can cause a surge of biochemical imbalances to occur within the body, including the disruption of the hypothalamus-pituitary axis, which can affect thyroid function and adrenal health. Intense cardio with little to no recovery time can all cause stress to the body, particularly thyroid function. For example, a sign of adrenal issues may be trying to exercise, only to find that you crash, feel light-headed and faint.

Cortisol will always be produced when we exercise, this is very normal, however, what we need to be aware of is if exercise is causing too much to be produced, due to our body feeling very stressed. To know this, we have to pay attention to our body following exercise.

If you experience heart palpitations, dizziness, back pain or any other worrying signs during pregnancy, stop and speak to your doctor. You'll need to be assessed for possible causes, while also reassessing if that type, frequency or intensity of exercise is still working for you at this point in pregnancy. Do not force exercise when you're experiencing anything like this.

We are all different and whereas some thyroid patients can maintain all forms of exercise throughout pregnancy, others cannot. If we overexert ourselves, it can inhibit thyroid function and contribute to adrenal stress, which can make pregnancy feel even more exhausting.

So, give yourself space to rediscover your happy place within exercise and movement. Starting from scratch if you're really fatigued in pregnancy may be necessary as well as ditching any preconceptions of what your exercise routine 'should' look like. Let your body tell you.

In general, exercise that has a risk of falling, including hockey, horse riding, gymnastics and cycling, are not advised during pregnancy. Exercise that involves lying flat on your back for long periods of time is also not advised, especially from 16 weeks onwards, because of the extra weight on the main blood vessel that is important for blood being brought back to your heart.

Try New Things

Pay attention to how different types of exercise make you feel and avoid doing types of exercise just because you think you 'should' be doing them.

Signs that you may need to reevaluate your exercise regimen during pregnancy:

- Fatigue that is long-lasting
- Thyroid flares following exercise
- Big blood sugar dips after working out
- Feeling muscle weakness and shakiness after working out

- Disrupted sleep
- Brain fog or cognitive issues
- Feeling worse after working out instead of more energised
- You cannot hold a conversation while exercising
- You feel out of breath

Exercise options that tend to be particularly popular among pregnant thyroid patients include yoga, swimming and walking. However, the best exercise is one that *you* enjoy and works for *your* body. Avoid any exercise that is clearly hindering you, worsening your health, makes any of your thyroid symptoms worse, or is feeling too intensive. As well as the type of exercise, consider how often your body is happy to do it, too. Some days you may feel up to walking and on less-energetic days some yoga stretches may help your body more, especially if certain pregnancy symptoms are more prevalent on certain days. Ideally, you want to be promoting more energy instead of only draining yourself further, as pregnancy is already tiring. Always increase intensity and frequency slowly and if your body struggles, please do listen to it.

It is obviously crucial to mention here that every person (and every thyroid patient) will be different. We will all have different needs when it comes to exercise, from type of exercise to frequency and intensity. You may well need to experiment with different types and frequencies to see what does and does not work for your body.

The time of day can also impact when you exercise. If you find that your blood sugar levels are affected or you have cortisol issues (many of us feel at our worst in the morning), you may find it better to exercise later on in the day, such as at lunchtime or in the afternoon.

I personally loved pregnancy yoga from around 13 weeks up until I gave birth and I even used a lot of poses and breathing techniques taught in class, *for* my birth. Most pregnancy yoga classes are so much more than just yoga. They tend to incorporate breathing techniques, hypnobirthing techniques, practising birthing positions and meditation. I would leave class feeling so calm and relaxed!

I also walked most days throughout both pregnancies, often for around 30-60 minutes a day. As I got further along in them, I experienced some pelvic girdle pain and sciatic pain which would make it difficult, so the walks got shorter the more pregnant I got. But I did love how adaptable walking was.

I enjoyed swimming for the 'weightless' feel it gave my bump, reducing back pain, overall aches and heaviness. As swimming is also very adaptable, you can do as much or as little as you feel is right.

Strength training is safe to continue in pregnancy as long as you feel well enough and have correct form. It is not recommended to take up a new type of exercise during pregnancy, but continuing with strength training can be very beneficial in keeping your body strong, as well as making labour and the postpartum period easier. It can reduce the chances of back pain following pregnancy. Strength training can also help manage blood sugar levels for those with type 2 or gestational diabetes. However, run it by your doctor in case it's not safe in your situation. For example, balance can become compromised as you progress through pregnancy, which can make you more prone to injury.

Be Kind to Yourself

When I was pregnant, I often found myself feeling guilty and ashamed that I wasn't exercising as much as I used to and wanted to. However, your body will not always be able to do exactly the same thing every single day. There are so many factors that can change day to day, from which stage of pregnancy you are in and what your body is focusing energy on that day, to how well you have slept, how nutritiously you have eaten, what other jobs are on your list for the day and how mentally drained you feel. As well as how your thyroid condition is doing during pregnancy. You're not going to feel up to exercising if you're feeling dreadful. Give yourself some flexibility and respect your body enough to know when to listen to it and follow its lead.

Get The Right Gear

When pregnant and exercising, you'll need a supportive, non-wired bra (most exercise bras are non-wired anyway), loose fitting tops and elasticated, loose trousers, along with supportive shoes. Use a yoga mat for yoga to avoid slipping, and if you're keen to swim, look at a maternity swimming costume that can be worn for the duration of your pregnancy if not also beyond.

Managing Expectations

Being pregnant, and especially when pregnant with health conditions such as hypothyroidism and Hashimoto's, can mean feeling less than fabulous. During my pregnancies, I understandably felt quite tired, fatigued and achy on some days. The first trimester was the hardest and as a result, I saw a sharp decline in my exercise activity. My two-weekly aerobic dance workouts became far too tiring to maintain, so I instead focused on walking and yoga.

There was a time in my early thyroid disease days, when I was only just diagnosed with hypothyroidism and Hashimoto's, that I would push my body to do more than it safely could, exercise-wise. Despite feeling exhausted, achy and lightheaded, I would force myself to do gym workouts and heavy cardio because I told myself that I was lazy if I did not. Realising that this was making my thyroid condition worse and adapting to a different type of exercise routine was crucial when recovering from and managing my autoimmune Hypothyroidism.

There were inevitably times in my pregnancies when I couldn't safely exercise, due to heavy fatigue and other symptoms, but when I skipped the session, those feelings of 'you're lazy' came flooding back to me. However, I distinctly remember one pregnancy yoga class I attended, around 5 months pregnant, where I made myself go, even though I felt borderline thyroid flarey that day. Half an hour into the class and I was suddenly very lightheaded and feeling funny. I started seeing spots in my vision and suddenly felt as if I was going to pass out.

I had to embarrassingly run out of the room and outside, where I took deep belly breaths in the fresh December air. It was the first time in my pregnancy that I felt so unwell when exercising and I realised that even yoga can be a workout on a pregnant body and especially one with preexisting health conditions! So, I unapologetically skipped class the following week as I was even more fatigued, achy and brain fogged and knew it wouldn't be wise to push myself so far past what my body could comfortably do. Please learn from my mistakes!

End of Chapter Checklist:

- ☐ I have the right exercising clothes for pregnancy.
- ☐ I am constantly reassessing my current exercise - type, frequency and intensity - and am listening to my body.
- ☐ I have tried pregnancy yoga and swimming.
- ☐ I am raising any concerns about exercise in pregnancy with my doctor.
- ☐ I am resting enough in between exercise sessions.
- ☐ I am listening to my body and not pushing exercise when I shouldn't.

Chapter 6: Your Healthcare Team in Pregnancy

There is a range of medical professionals you may see during pregnancy with thyroid disease and you are definitely not alone if you're confused about it all! Should you see a GP / PCP, endocrinologist, obstetrician and what on Earth is a midwife?!

First of all, let's look at the difference between:

Mainstream Medicine and Functional Medicine

There are generally two approaches to medicine, conventional / mainstream medicine and functional medicine (also known as: lifestyle medicine, integrative, progressive, alternative medicine and holistic medicine).

Mainstream medicine is what many of us are most familiar with. It follows the conventional ways a doctor treats a patient. For example, someone presents with a symptom or problem and they're given a drug to help with that. Functional medicine looks at getting to the root cause of the symptoms, and fixing that, before going straight to treating the symptom/s with drugs, as well as looking at your whole lifestyle (diet, stress, exercise and much more).

For many people, conventional medicine works just fine for them in pregnancy, whereas for others, they feel that a functional medicine approach is better suited to them and their needs. For example, as I was on NDT medication, a treatment not routinely used by the NHS, I needed and benefited from the monitoring and management of a functional doctor too.

Functional practitioners are also interested in whether your hypothyroidism is autoimmune, whereas mainstream medicine is less concerned about this. Due to cost restraints, mainstream medicine doctors may not be able to use more innovative tests and treatments and often cannot spend enough time to help identify, run tests or treat complex autoimmune diseases and hormonal imbalances. They also tend to have longer waiting times and more rushed appointments. Saying all of this, many, many people utilise mainstream maternity care (in the UK we have the NHS for example) and are very happy with their care. It really can be personal to you and your health situation, including your thyroid condition and how well that is managed, during pregnancy.

You may find that seeing just the one type of doctor or practitioner works for you, however, combining the expertise of more than one can also be useful. This is known as having a 'healthcare team' look after you.

Your pregnancy healthcare team may be made up of:

- A GP / PCP – either on the NHS, private or covered by insurance
- A Midwife
- An Endocrinologist
- A Functional Medicine Doctor / Functional Medicine Practitioner
- A Naturopathic Doctor / Naturopathic Practitioner
- An Obstetrician

- A Mental Health Therapist
- A Doula

We'll look at each of these in more detail, including why they may be a useful part of your team.

GP or PCP

GP stands for 'general practitioner', PCP stands for 'primary care provider'. These medical doctors are not specialists in a particular area or field and as such, tend to know a standard amount about all aspects of the body, rather than being focused on one area or system alone.

Most, if not all of us, will have a GP or PCP make up part of our healthcare team during pregnancy by default.

Midwife

Common in the UK and a few other countries too (Canada, Australia, New Zealand, Abu Dhabi), midwives are health professionals who care for women in pregnancy, labour and the first month or two after birth. For countries that use them, they are usually the first port of call for pregnant women and take the lead on their care. If your pregnancy is deemed low risk and straightforward, you may *only* see a midwife for the duration of your pregnancy.

Community midwives look after pregnant women up until they enter hospital to give birth, whereby a hospital midwife then takes over their care. After giving birth and returning home, a community midwife usually takes over again. Whereas hospital midwives only work in the hospital, community midwives may visit you at home, in doctor's clinics or other family centres.

They will check in with you over regular appointments, measure your bump, blood pressure, listen to the baby's heartbeat and advise on breastfeeding support, birth options and more. They do not perform surgery or practise medicine, so are not doctors and cannot issue prescriptions, but they will refer you to your usual doctor / GP if anything is out of their remit.

It is not common for your first midwife appointment to occur before 8 weeks of pregnancy here in the UK. I saw the midwife for the first time in both pregnancies around 8-9 weeks. This was a bit of a shock to me to find that you have your first antenatal appointment a good month after finding out you are pregnant!

Doula

A doula can be a great support to pregnant, labouring and postpartum women. Providing practical and emotional support, they are a non-medical professional who can be a valuable voice for you during pregnancy and birth. Doulas will not deliver your baby, instead they aim to complement the care of midwives, obstetricians and other doctors. Doulas will ensure that you are looked after and comfortable, and that your wishes are clearly advocated for. They will guide you through pregnancy, birth and post-partum, with their focus being on supporting the mother-to-be and the transition for her and baby during labour. If you would like to explore the addition of a doula, please research their background, experience, testimonies and whether they are a fit for you and your beliefs and values.

Endocrinologist

An endocrinologist specialises in the endocrine system. A referral to an endocrinologist can be made by your usual doctor. Endocrinologists are somewhat of a controversial topic among thyroid patients. Whereas some find a good level of success with an endocrinologist during pregnancy, others feel that they follow mainstream medicine "too closely" and thus, do not offer much more than their GP or PCP. However, if your pregnancy is more high risk, an endocrinologist may be involved in your care.

Depending on where you are in the world, endocrinologists can offer more than T4-only medication but often only prefer to prescribe conventional T4 synthetics during pregnancy.

Private GP or Private Doctor

Private doctors in the UK mostly fall into mainstream medicine but often offer more than NHS GPs. For example, the NHS only offers the thyroid medication Levothyroxine for the most part, but private doctors may offer more types of thyroid medication in pregnancy. They are often keen to do more in-depth and comprehensive testing, such as the full thyroid panel, too.

Functional Medicine Doctor or Functional Medicine Practitioner

Functional medicine doctors and functional medicine practitioners offer more comprehensive testing than mainstream doctors, look at optimising other aspects of your life, including diet, routines for sleeping and stress coping, and prefer to treat by looking at the whole body as a system that needs to work in harmony together, rather than focusing on the thyroid gland alone.

Not all functional practitioners have medical degrees, so whilst some are Functional Medicine Doctors, others are simply Functional Medicine Practitioners. Many thyroid patients around the world will utilise a functional medicine doctor / practitioner alongside a mainstream doctor, as it can be useful to implement knowledge and practises from both.

Naturopath or Naturopathic Doctor

A naturopath applies natural therapies to health conditions, often to complement what you're receiving from a conventional or functional doctor. This includes dietary changes, lifestyle changes, acupuncture and herbal medicine for example.

They provide personalised care to each patient, and, similarly to a functional medicine practitioner, see the body as a holistic unity of body, mind, and spirit, aiming to address the body as one.

They usually practice in a freelance environment, but have the option to work in hospitals, spas and healthcare, too. Not all naturopaths have medical degrees, so whilst some are Naturopathic Doctors, others are simply Naturopaths. Only those with medical degrees can write prescriptions such as those for thyroid medications. Just like functional medicine doctors and practitioners, you would usually pay privately to see a naturopath.

Obstetricians

Obstetricians can also help to manage thyroid conditions during pregnancy. These specialists are generally concerned with the care of a pregnant woman, her unborn child and the management of diseases specific to women, such as thyroid issues, which can come to light during pregnancy, be triggered by pregnancy or get worse during pregnancy.

Many practitioners in this field have a special interest in one particular area, such as high-risk obstetrics, fertility care or minimal access surgery.

You can be referred to an obstetrician when pregnant by your GP in the UK. However, in the US, obstetricians and OB-GYNS are often the primary lead on antenatal care.

Therapist

A therapist can be useful if you experience mental health effects such as depression or anxiety during pregnancy. These mental health conditions can be directly caused by a thyroid condition or pregnancy hormones, as well as made worse by or simply triggered by them.

Counselling, cognitive behavioural therapy, as well as other options are available when it comes to talking about juggling your pregnancy and thyroid health, as well as other things.

Many people find that having a mental health professional in their healthcare team is of huge help and support when navigating health conditions and pregnancy.

So, who is the best practitioner to manage you in pregnancy?

I wish I could tell you! I hope this chapter has at least educated you on your options and who you may meet while pregnant.

End of Chapter Checklist:

- ☐ I have booked an appointment with my doctor, midwife, etc.
- ☐ I understand my options for medical professionals during pregnancy.
- ☐ I have considered which types of doctors and medical professionals I would like involved in my pregnancy with thyroid disease.
- ☐ I have all current appointments noted down in my calendar.
- ☐ I have any questions I wish to ask noted down.

Chapter 7: Rachel's Pregnancies (and how they were so different!)

When you embark on pregnancy as someone with a health condition, you definitely have an inkling that it could be quite different to a 'regular healthy person's'. However, I didn't expect my own two pregnancies to be so wildly different.

This chapter is not as informational as others. It delves into the specifics of my own pregnancies with thyroid disease and how and why they differed, so it is much more a retelling of my personal experiences. I also cover the expectations and preconceptions I had of going into pregnancy with a thyroid condition and on unconventional medication, and whether they came true or not.

Round 1

In the summer of 2019, I found out I was expecting my first child and I was over the moon. It wasn't a huge surprise as they had been long hoped for and wanted more than anything in the world. I pretty much had the pregnancy you see in films; I was glowing, it was straightforward and fairly textbook.

At the time of falling pregnant, all thyroid levels were optimal and I was in great health. My Hashimoto's was also in remission. I was on NDT medication called Armour Thyroid.

I confirmed my pregnancy at 4 weeks, just a day before my period was due. Overall, I felt quite tired during the first trimester, and even wondered if it was down to my thyroid condition as it felt just like thyroid fatigue. However, blood tests showed that my thyroid levels were good, so it must have been general pregnancy fatigue.

I saw the private GP (who prescribes my Armour Thyroid) when I was 5 weeks pregnant and he had no issues at all with me carrying on this medication during pregnancy. He didn't want to increase the dose immediately but rather wait for blood test results which he would receive a week later. My levels were already optimal at a recent test and he didn't want to risk overmedicating me. He also printed out some information for me to pass to my NHS GP regarding why he would be favouring Free T3 and Free T4 levels over TSH alone while managing me during pregnancy.

My NHS GP appointment (also at 5 weeks pregnant) went well too, and better than expected. I was anxious about him pushing back about the Armour Thyroid, but he actually acknowledged that some people do not do well on Levothyroxine. So, he was happy for me to continue the Armour Thyroid during pregnancy and mainly be managed by the private GP, but did make a referral to an NHS endocrinologist and obstetrician to get their input.

The NHS GP explained that I would need a full thyroid panel checking every 4 to 6 weeks during pregnancy. I was pleased that he was so on the ball with testing my levels often, as it meant I saved a lot of money from ordering them myself, privately. My first thyroid test was at 5 weeks pregnant and the results came back with my thyroid levels still optimal, but I asked the private GP if I could increase my dose slightly to support the development in the first trimester (see Chapter 4). He agreed for me to increase it ever so slightly and then be retested in another 4 to 6 weeks or so, but if I felt unwell at any time, he suggested I lower it again and be tested sooner.

At 8 weeks pregnant, I decided to have a private ultrasound scan (with Ultrasound Direct - booked online) to calm my anxiety about a small amount of bleeding I was experiencing, and the baby was measuring 'perfect' in size and heart rate, which was a huge relief.

My first midwife appointment at 8 weeks was very positive. She was more than happy to leave the 'thyroid stuff' to the GPs, and couldn't see any reason for me to be a high risk pregnancy. I was really happy.

Also at 8 weeks, I had my first appointment with the NHS endocrinologist and, as expected, the endocrinologist lectured me about being on Armour Thyroid medication and told me that if it wasn't prescribed, i.e. self-sourced (which I used to do before obtaining it on private prescription) then she would have to make me go back to Levothyroxine. I have since learned however, that this is incorrect as no medical professional can force any type of treatment on you during pregnancy.

As my Armour Thyroid *is* prescribed, she said she couldn't suggest much in terms of managing this during pregnancy but could only recommend that I move back to Levothyroxine, despite both me and my husband explaining in detail to her how ill I was on Levothyroxine. She suggested that my low TSH (which is often seen as 'normal' with NDT) and being on Armour Thyroid in pregnancy was not safe and could cause issues such as miscarriage and other risks.

I asked to be discharged and she agreed that there was nothing she could add to the situation. At 10 weeks, I had my second set of thyroid tests. They showed that I was now slightly overmedicated, so both the NHS and private GP suggested I lower my Armour Thyroid dosage back to the original amount, which I did (and also agreed with). I booked a further private ultrasound scan at 10 weeks due to a bit more bleeding, but all was fine still.

I saw the NHS GP again at 12 weeks to discuss how I was getting on. After the endocrinologist discharged me a few weeks prior, the NHS GP said that he was happy to leave it at that and that he was glad an endocrinologist had at least had the opportunity to be involved.

I had my first NHS ultrasound scan at 13 weeks, which showed that everything was developing normally. I had a same day appointment with an obstetrician, which my GP had referred me to due to being on unconventional thyroid medication. However, she had no cause for concern and didn't see my hypothyroidism, Hashimoto's or NDT as a specific risk factor in the pregnancy, but did want to monitor me closely to make sure the private GP was dosing the NDT correctly.

I developed itchy hands and a rash at 13 weeks, making my wedding and engagement ring tighter. A blood test came back with mildly elevated AST and ALT levels (liver enzymes), so a same day appointment with the GP was made by my midwife, but they weren't overly concerned. I was told I had mild intrahepatic cholestasis of pregnancy. My AST and ALT levels were checked every 6 to 8 weeks throughout pregnancy from this point and they dropped back into normal range towards the end. Another thyroid test at 14 weeks, 18 weeks and 23 weeks all showed that my thyroid levels were still optimal and I still did not require an increase in Armour Thyroid medication dosage.

The anatomy scan was performed at 19 weeks, where everything looked perfect and the baby was even measuring a little ahead of their due date. We also found out it was a boy. The obstetrician saw me again at this appointment and had nothing else to add. Happy with the private GP handling my thyroid, she discharged me, recommending that the NHS GP was to keep testing my thyroid levels every month throughout pregnancy. I also had my flu and whooping cough vaccines, with no issues to report.

At 29 weeks, I had another thyroid blood test. The results showed that my Free T4 was only just within range and my Free T3 had dropped too. Being on NDT medication, my TSH was suppressed, as expected. Both the NHS GP and private GP agreed that an increase in my medication was finally needed, so we raised the dosage and then retested in another 4 weeks' time. Before now, I hadn't needed any dosage increase at all.

The results came back and showed that my levels were now optimal again, however, my Iron levels came back low at this point, so I started an Iron supplement. I took Bisglycinate as it's easy on the stomach. I had another midwife check-up at 31 weeks, which showed that my liver test results were still coming back normal. At 34 weeks, we had another completely normal and positive check-up appointment.

At 35 weeks, I ended up having another extra ultrasound scan after having a fall at home. Besides my bruised knees and sciatica, I was OK and the baby was too. The scan confirmed he was measuring 2 weeks ahead still and was a very healthy weight. This was reassuring to hear as a thyroid patient. At 35 weeks I also had another Iron and liver test which came back good. My third trimester was progressing very smoothly, with no concerns from anyone.

I had another routine midwife appointment at 36 weeks. The baby was measuring on-time and everything was looking good. I had opted for a birth at a midwife-led unit from the beginning and was on track to have this due to having a non-high risk and uncomplicated pregnancy so far. Another routine midwife appointment at 38 weeks and 6 days was also all positive.

From 34 weeks, I experienced a few thyroid flares due to overcommitting myself and agreeing to too many social events. I made the decision to prioritise being at home and resting whenever possible from then on.

I gave birth at 39 weeks, with labour starting on its own. My birth is covered in the next chapter.

Pregnancy ailments I experienced included heartburn, sciatic pain towards the end (a pregnancy pillow and exercise ball helped though), itchy skin (from intrahepatic cholestasis), leg cramps, nausea (but not sickness thankfully) and I felt ravenous all the time in the first trimester!

Round 2

In the autumn of 2021, I found out I was expecting again, and once again, it was hoped for and I tested before my period was even due (I was excited, ok?!)

This pregnancy was less textbook, less straightforward and there was **no** glowing! Compared to being on Armour Thyroid NDT for my first pregnancy, my second saw me on Armour alongside Levothyroxine, an adjustment I'd made a year before, when my firstborn was six months old and my body's needs had changed. However, with this being my second pregnancy, I was more confident that I could indeed have a healthy pregnancy and baby at the end and that I knew which bumps I may come up against.

I was overall less anxious about navigating pregnancy with Hypothyroidism, Hashimoto's and privately prescribed Armour and Levothyroxine. At the time of falling pregnant, I was on 150mg Armour Thyroid and 25mcg Levothyroxine. All thyroid levels (TSH, Free T3, Free T4, thyroid peroxidase antibodies and thyroglobulin antibodies) were optimal and I was in great health. My Hashimoto's was still in remission.

I spoke to the private GP for the first time during this pregnancy when I was 4 weeks pregnant. He was very happy for me and had no issues with me carrying on the NDT and

Levothyroxine combination during pregnancy at all. He said that as long as I felt well and blood tests taken regularly looked optimal, then we could carry on. We planned to manage my thyroid medication in the same way we had done with the first pregnancy; testing my TSH, Free T3 and Free T4 every 4-6 weeks and then monitoring these to make adjustments as necessary.

My NHS GP appointment (also at 4 weeks pregnant) went well too. I was still with the same NHS GP as my first pregnancy over two years before, and he remembered it well. He had no concerns this time around and said that unlike last time, he didn't see a need to refer me to an endocrinologist or obstetrician as he was confident I would be fine again.

The NHS GP agreed with my private GP on needing to test the full thyroid panel every 4 to 6 weeks throughout pregnancy and that my private doctor could use these results too, to save us running more tests than was necessary

I booked in for my first thyroid blood test and had it taken at 5 weeks pregnant. The results came back with my thyroid levels still optimal so we kept medication dosage the same for now. The midwife referral was also made for when I was 9 weeks pregnant. I would have my next set of bloods taken at this too.

At 7 weeks pregnant, I had a private ultrasound scan, to calm anxiety about a small amount of bleeding I had (something I experienced in both pregnancies). The baby was measuring well and the heartbeat was strong, which was a huge relief.

My first midwife appointment went well; she didn't bat an eye at my thyroid medication. I had my blood drawn again at 9 weeks pregnant, and they came back a few days later, with a change. My Free T4 had now dropped to the bottom of the range although my Free T3 had barely moved. Both the NHS and private GPs agreed that an increase in Levothyroxine was needed. I went from 150mg Armour + 25mcg Levothyroxine to 150mg Armour + 50mcg Levothyroxine. Within a few weeks I was feeling much better.

My first NHS ultrasound scan was performed at 12 weeks which showed that everything was going well and the baby was developing perfectly. I had my thyroid levels checked again at 13 weeks. Just as with my first pregnancy, they were being tested every 4 weeks. However, we were all surprised to see that when we retested my levels at 13 weeks, 4 weeks after the dosage increase, they hadn't really moved. We all decided to wait a couple more weeks, to allow the change in medication some more time to 'finish building' in my blood and retest.

However, during these weeks, I felt dreadful. I was heavily fatigued the entire time; my eyelashes were falling out and I was depressed. Thyroid fatigue is unlike anything else. I was dragging myself around in a haze, everything moving slowly and fuzzily. I was quite depressed around this time. I knew I needed more thyroid hormone replacement medication.

So, we retested and my free T4 was still low within range, despite the recent medication increase. We upped my Levothyroxine again, to 75mcg, alongside the original 150mg of Armour. Testing my levels another 4 weeks later, so at this point, 18 weeks pregnant, the Free T4 had finally moved back to the middle of the range, which is what my doctor considers optimised. Within a week I was feeling completely better.

My thyroid levels for this pregnancy were proving to be more unpredictable than my first, moving around often and suddenly plummeting multiple times.

At around 18 weeks, I also self-arranged some vitamin testing to check which supplements I still needed (resources for this are included at the end of this book). My Vitamin D was excellent but my Ferritin was on the low end of normal. Increasing my supplementation of Iron Bisglycinate helped a lot.

At 14 weeks, we heard the baby's heartbeat for the first time at a midwife appointment and all was developing well. However, we received some delayed news from the hospital following some non-thyroid related blood test results, which informed me of two complications found in my pregnancy which would put me in the 'high risk' category.

This news was a shock to receive and process. I was told that the abnormal liver levels from the first pregnancy had returned (except not so mild this time) and that I had intrahepatic cholestasis of pregnancy, as well as Low Papp-A, a condition found in around 5% of pregnancies which indicates that the placenta may not work very well. Both of these conditions meant that I would have extra blood tests and ultrasound scans throughout my pregnancy to monitor the baby more closely, as my risk for premature labour, stillbirth and more all increased. All new to me, after a straightforward and non-high risk first pregnancy, I felt really daunted, even though I was reassured that most women who experience these issues are fine.

I had a scan at 16 weeks, which showed that everything was normal with the baby's development so far, and we also discovered I was carrying another son.

At 20 weeks, the NHS anatomy scan again confirmed that so far, everything was looking absolutely perfect. I also had my flu and whooping cough vaccines, with no issues to report.

I had some thyroid flare days during my second trimester, but they were very brief and I didn't experience as many as I did during the first trimester. They mainly occurred around the time my thyroid levels kept dropping.

At 21 weeks I had a telephone appointment with an NHS obstetrician about the factors that made my pregnancy high risk. She explained that so far, everything was tracking fine, so it was a case of hoping this was the trend as we kept moving forward.

At 22 weeks, I spent an evening at the hospital being screened for pre-eclampsia (which was eventually ruled out) after having slightly high blood pressure and an ongoing headache for 5 days.

The bloods I had taken at 27 weeks came back when I was 28 weeks pregnant and showed that my thyroid levels were still optimal, with my Free T4 midrange and Free T3 in the top quarter of the range. Both the NHS GP and Private GP were happy with this. I also felt well, i.e. no thyroid symptoms at this point.

A thyroid blood test was repeated at 32 weeks pregnant, which also came back with levels optimal still and having not moved. I was having my thyroid panel checked every month throughout pregnancy and ultrasounds scans performed every month too.

Midwife appointments were happening every 2-3 weeks at this point and going well. No concerns were had and the midwife was happy with everything. The baby was incredibly active and already head down by 30 weeks.

I didn't experience any thyroid flare days during the third trimester but did feel overall more tired.

At 34 weeks, I experienced a preterm labour scare after I caught a vomiting bug which quickly dehydrated me so much that it triggered contractions and I was sent to the hospital to be assessed. Midwives and doctors acted quickly and halted the contractions and I stayed in hospital for three days before being cleared to go home, as long as I agreed to "not overdo things".

At 36 weeks, the obstetrician discharged me and put me back to being midwife led and no longer 'high risk', based on the growth scans and other tests and vitals being consistently good. This was fabulous news. I was also told I could have the midwife unit birth I had hoped for, after spending the whole pregnancy unsure if this would be the case or if I'd have to have a hospital labour suite birth.

My last thyroid blood test was taken at 37 weeks. My Free T4 had once again fallen suddenly below range, with my Free T3 still optimal. My Levothyroxine dose was therefore increased again, making my final thyroid medication combination: 150mg Armour Thyroid + 100mcg Levothyroxine. I had begun the pregnancy on 150mg Armour Thyroid + 25mcg Levothyroxine.

I can't stress enough how important it is to have thyroid levels checked often in pregnancy. Having mine checked every 4 weeks meant we caught any sudden drops in thyroid hormone very quickly.

My midwife appointments at 35 and 37 weeks went well, with normal blood pressure noted, exams showing the baby was head down and 'engaged' and a normal foetal heartbeat. I gave birth at 38 weeks, with labour starting on its own again. More in the next chapter on this.

As you can see, this was a more eventful pregnancy and I felt as if I couldn't breathe until I received that call at 37 weeks to reassure me that the 'high risk' status was no longer required.

Pregnancy ailments I experienced this time around included heartburn, sciatic pain, 'morning sickness' (but I was always throwing up around midnight), hot flushes, cramps in my hands at night and insomnia.

Were My Pregnancies as a Thyroid Patient What I Expected?

Like a lot of people living with a thyroid condition, I had worries and concerns surrounding a pregnancy with hypothyroidism and Hashimoto's. Add in that I'm on unconventional thyroid medication and I certainly had a lot of thoughts and expectations surrounding what it may be like. Did my expectations come true?

Unsurprisingly, it was a mixed bag in that regard. I'll talk about some of the expectations I had that *did* come true first.

The first was that being pregnant on NDT medication would involve a lot of arguing with medical professionals about this. The NHS does not routinely prescribe anything other than Levothyroxine and therefore, is not massively familiar with managing NDT medication. Especially so in pregnant individuals! I expected to be explaining why I was on this medication at every medical appointment, needing to justify it constantly and continually putting my foot down about not going back onto Levothyroxine in place of it. In general, I thought there would be a big push to take my NDT away and that the NHS doctors would disagree with the private doctor who prescribes it. I was worried that after feeling so much pressure to do so, the private doctor may well pull out of prescribing me the NDT.

During my first son's pregnancy, I was referred to an endocrinologist who did their best to convince me to change back to Levothyroxine during pregnancy, but after I declined, they discharged me and left the managing of my thyroid medication to the private GP. From that point onwards, no other medical professional I experienced during either of my pregnancies raised it again. That initial appointment with the endocrinologist was stressful but they didn't push it beyond that discussion.

Another expectation I had that came true was an increase in thyroid flare days, expecting the pregnancy to exacerbate my Hashimoto's and thyroid symptoms. I also expected my thyroid levels to move around a lot during pregnancy, as my thyroid condition would become less 'stable' due to the effects and demands of pregnancy on the thyroid gland. During my first son's pregnancy, I experienced more flares, but not a lot. My thyroid levels were also very stable and easily managed.

However, during the second, I had more flares and my thyroid levels were much less stable. My medication needed adjusting multiple times as levels changed dramatically and suddenly. Luckily, I was having thyroid blood tests every month throughout both pregnancies, which meant we caught any changes quickly.

The third expectation I had was that I would have to fight to have the full thyroid panel checked during pregnancy (as explained in Chapter 3, this is important). When I informed my NHS GP of the pregnancy, I made it clear that I would require at the very least TSH, Free T3 and Free T4 to be checked every 4-6 weeks. He said that he was onboard to check these levels every 4-6 weeks, not least because of the type of thyroid medication I was taking, which contained T3 and required us to check Free T3 and Free T4 to ensure correct dosing of it. Had he not agreed to this, I would have budgeted to pay for these extra tests myself from somewhere like Medichecks or LetsGetChecked, which I already use for extra testing when working with my private doctor (listed at the back of this book). I did have to remind all midwives, nurses and doctors that I required the full thyroid panel to be checked every time and not just TSH.

My fourth expectation was that I would have multiple doctors involved in my pregnancies. I expected a lot of specialists and consultants to be involved due to taking NDT medication, however, this didn't really happen. Instead, they were involved a lot due to the other complications and risk factors.

The fifth on this list is that my migraines would get worse and also that I wouldn't be able to take Sumatriptan for them. I am prescribed this medication for migraines I get around my period and suspected that I may get more migraines with the hormonal fluctuations of pregnancy. I experienced a few during the first trimester of each pregnancy, but none thereafter, and I was indeed right in that Sumatriptan is not recommended in pregnancy. My doctor advised that I should avoid taking sumatriptan if possible, because they don't know whether it could have adverse effects on a pregnancy. In the end, I managed the migraines without sumatriptan, although they were very painful.

The sixth expectation that came true on this list is that I would have a lot of extra blood tests. All doctors involved in my care agreed that I needed regular, full thyroid panel blood tests throughout pregnancy. When not pregnant, my thyroid levels are tested every 6 months, so going from this to once a month was definitely a big increase in the amount of blood draws! My midwife also decided to run other regular tests too, including those for diabetes, liver function and vitamin levels such as Ferritin and Vitamin D, due to my thyroid condition. On average, I was having blood tests every couple of weeks all the way through my pregnancies.

Another expectation that came true was that I may be classed as a 'High Risk Pregnancy'. Not all pregnant people with a thyroid condition will automatically be classed as high risk. It is decided on a patient by patient basis and factors such as which type of thyroid medication you are on, how well controlled your thyroid condition is and whether you have other risk factors will impact this. (All explained in Chapter 4)

In terms of the expectations I had prior to pregnancy that did *not* come true, the main one was probably that I would struggle to fall pregnant, which I was very fortunate to not experience. I fell pregnant quickly all three times. How much of that was due to the steps I incorporated from Chapter 3? I'll never know for sure. Many thyroid patients struggle to fall pregnant (which is why I wrote this book). After years of my periods being really heavy, irregular and I wasn't even ovulating, I was unsure if I'd even be able to fall pregnant at all, let alone 'easily'. Doctors also warned me that having thyroid disease could impact whether I'd be able to fall and stay pregnant one day.

I also thought I would feel worse when pregnant but overall, I had the opposite. Minus the typical pregnancy symptoms of fatigue, sickness and aches and pains, I felt better while pregnant in terms of my thyroid condition, in my first pregnancy. I experienced less flares, my Hashimoto's stayed in remission and undetectable for both pregnancies, and my thyroid symptoms were non-existent as long as my thyroid levels were kept in the optimal range (which is why testing them so often was important). Thyroid symptoms I had previous to pregnancy, such as acne, hugely improved while pregnant.

I also thought I would need a lot of thyroid medication dosage adjustments. This was not true for my first pregnancy.

I was on Armour Thyroid for the first, the dose of which remained constant and kept my thyroid levels optimal right until the last two months of pregnancy. It surprised us all, since most need a medication dosage alteration before this! It was increased by just 15% for the last two months.

In my second pregnancy, the Armour Thyroid did not need adjusting, but the Levothyroxine I was on alongside it was different. This was adjusted two times during the first 20 weeks alone and once more towards the end of pregnancy.

Another expectation I had was that I could continue my pre-pregnancy exercise. Prior to my first pregnancy, I did a mix of exercise, however, by the time I was in the second trimester of my first pregnancy, I found that I could no longer safely keep up with it. I was feeling lightheaded and therefore needed to reassess.

My Babies Were Healthy

Thankfully, my two baby boys arrived healthy and without any issues. Looking back now at the Rachel who was so very anxious at the thought of having children because she wasn't sure if she'd be able to have them or get through pregnancy with all the thyroid luggage, I would love to reassure her that it *can* be done and that it has been *so worth it.*

Yes, having hypothyroidism and / or Hashimoto's does indeed increase the chances of pregnancy loss and other complications, however, much of this can be avoided with correct monitoring and management. I feel incredibly lucky for my children and of course, I appreciate that not everyone has the same experience, but I hope that my experiences can bring some reassurance to those who have similar anxieties too.

Chapter 8: Giving Birth

Planning your birth is a very personal experience. What I will start off by saying is this:

Think of it less as a 'Birth Plan' and more of a 'Birth Preference'.

This simple change can really impact how you view this part of the process. You see, assuming we can plan *every* detail of our birth gives us a false sense of control, and should your labour and birth not follow your plan exactly, it can lead to you feeling very out of control and disempowered by the experience. Our bodies are amazing. Birth is an incredible process that it goes through, but is it easy? Not for many. However, can we be prepared? Definitely.

For general labour and birth planning, I highly recommend the book *The Positive Birth Book* by Milli Hill. Honestly, it was the single best book I read to prepare me for labour and birth. It walks you through options for location (a hospital labour unit birth, midwife unit birth, home birth etc.), as well as medication (such as epidurals) and non-medication options for pain relief. It breaks down the different stages and made me feel so empowered before giving birth.

Using the book, I created birth plans for three possibilities: a midwife unit birth (my preference), a hospital labour unit birth (my Plan B) and an emergency C-Section. This way, whichever turn my births may have taken, I could feel that my wants and needs were being understood and met for all and any situation. Having the birth plans printed and in my hospital bag also meant that my husband could refer to them in case I was unable to make decisions myself. He knew he was following my wishes by referring to them as well. It empowered both of us.

I personally wanted a non-medical birth, but was not comfortable being at home for a few reasons, mainly because I liked the idea of being close to doctors if I did suddenly encounter an emergency with the birth. The midwife unit I used for both births was located inside a hospital, but I would be tended to by midwives only, in a cosy, low-lit and calming room. The hormone oxytocin, which is so important in progressing labour, prefers these environments. It did not feel clinical at all and this was what I wanted. The option of gas and air (Entonox) was available, but no epidural, which I was fine with. Had I been declared high-risk by the time I reached full term (37 weeks), the midwife led unit would not have been an option.

Both of my births were straightforward. I had midwife unit births with no medical interventions and using only gas and air. I know that, personally, my body tends to react or have the listed rare side effects to almost everything I take, so I chose to limit my pain relief due to this. You will know what feels best *for you*. I chose to focus on hypnobirthing techniques for pain relief and then also utilising gas and air when it felt necessary. I used birth pools to help relax me and for a calmer experience.

However, had they not gone to plan and I needed to be transferred or I felt that I did indeed want stronger pain relief, then my husband and I could refer back to the other preferences I had listed out. Nothing needed to be set in stone, but I entered my labours feeling prepared.

I am often asked about epidurals, which carry no extra risks for thyroid patients compared to non-thyroid patients, but they do carry an increased risk in a drop in blood pressure, back pain after birth, nausea, a slower delivery process and a higher risk of a forceps or ventouse-assisted delivery.

I was also hoping to avoid an induction, since these are linked with a higher chance of medical intervention being needed and was lucky that my labours both started on their own at 38 and 39 weeks with some mild contractions. There are many old wives tales around starting labour naturally - spicy food, pineapples, long walks, bumpy car rides, bouncing on a pregnancy ball, sex, etc. but none are proven to work. My labours both started after a walk, which perhaps helped.

While pregnant, I took a hypnobirthing course and practised the breathing and visualisation techniques throughout pregnancy and labour, which helped me with pain management and nurturing oxytocin. I also made music playlists on my phone; a calm playlist, a romantic playlist and a motivational playlist. I utilised each one at different points in labour, using the calm one towards the end, the motivational one early on and the romantic one when I needed a gentle slow dance with my husband to encourage a sense of calm, connection and oxytocin, to - you guessed it! - encourage straightforward labour that did not require interventions. With my knowledge in adrenal health, promoting helpful labour hormones and reducing stress hormones like cortisol, it made so much sense to me to promote low stress levels throughout pregnancy and labour. Learning some simple hypnobirthing techniques such as how to breath during labour in order to make it easier can go a long way.

It is advised to pack a hospital bag, which you can keep near your front door, ready to grab when labour starts. Having it packed and ready to go when you reach around 36 weeks of pregnancy is a good idea (though you can do it before, by all means!)

What I Included in my hospital bag:

- A few days' worth of thyroid medication (you may be in hospital for longer than you expect)
- Any other medications or essential supplements you take
- Spritz for Bits spray (amazing stuff – a natural spray formula created by midwives to soothe pain after childbirth)
- *The Positive Birth Book* (for referring to in labour)
- Snacks for labour to keep blood sugar up (cheese, nuts, protein bars)
- Water bottle
- Pregnancy notes and birth plan (several copies)
- Sponge for birth pool
- Changes of clothes (loose and comfy) (3 tops, 2 PJ bottoms)
- Breast pads
- Lip balm
- Lots of underwear
- Toothbrush
- Toothpaste
- Face wash cloth
- Body wash
- Shampoo
- Conditioner
- Deodorant
- Hair ties
- Face wash
- Face moisturiser
- Wash towel x1
- Labour Nightdress x2 (many women prefer giving birth in a loose pyjama dress)

- Paracetamol
- Clothes and nappies for baby
- Hair brush
- Massage oil for during labour (having a birth partner massage your lower back in labour can feel great)
- Phone charger
- Maternity pads for underwear
- Baby wipes
- That bouncy exercise ball from pregnancy! Excellent in labour!

After giving birth, I was instructed by the doctor to return to my pre-pregnancy thyroid medication dose immediately. Since you're already guaranteed to be exhausted following childbirth, making sure you support your body by packing any essential medication and supplements is important.

Sending you best wishes for an empowering birth experience!

End of Chapter Checklist:

- ☐ I have made a list for my hospital bag.
- ☐ I have packed my hospital bag!
- ☐ I have educated myself on what to expect for labour and options for location, pain management and more.
- ☐ I have made 'birth plans' / a birth preference sheet.
- ☐ I have discussed preferences with my midwife / doctor and confirmed where I am able to give birth.

Part Three: Taking Care of Yourself During Postpartum and Parenting

Chapter 9: What Does Thyroid Health Look Like After Pregnancy?

Before I ever fell pregnant, I often wondered (and worried) what pregnancy, childbirth and postpartum would do to my thyroid health.

Living with autoimmune hypothyroidism, my health could be up and down and, after having managed to get it stable for a couple of years, I started to think about starting my own family but remained curious about whether it would have any long lasting impact on my Hashimoto's and hypothyroidism.

Predicting what a thyroid patient's health is going to be like during pregnancy and after giving birth is nigh on impossible, but it doesn't mean you can't be prepared. Whereas some women with hypothyroidism report feeling better when pregnant, for many others, they feel worse and this can get worse following delivering their baby too, due to thyroid hormone levels needing time to settle back into place post-birth.

You can prepare for needing more support than the average person by building a support network prior to the baby's arrival, such as people you can count on to help cook meals, do laundry or otherwise help you out.

Thyroid hormone levels can take anywhere from a few weeks to a few months to iron out in women with hypothyroidism who have given birth, and this should be taken into consideration too. For some women, they may also benefit from seeing a functional medicine practitioner, naturopath or other progressive medicine practitioner, for addressing adrenal health, stress and holistic support following birth.

Maximising how much time the new parent with a thyroid issue gets to sleep, rest and recuperate will go a long way in getting their health back on track so they can be as conscious and present as possible.

What Will Happen to Your Thyroid Levels After Pregnancy?

What your thyroid levels do after pregnancy and in that postpartum period will be unique to you. Although the postpartum period can be tiring, difficult and an important time for recovery following pregnancy and childbirth, many find they do better than they had anticipated during this time.

After giving birth both times, I went back to my pre-pregnancy thyroid medication dosage immediately, had my levels tested 6 weeks later, found they were optimal and felt overall in good health (besides the sleep deprivation that a newborn brings!). I tested levels again at two months postpartum and they were the same. However, at around six months postpartum from my first child, thyroid antibodies went up, signalling that my Hashimoto's was out of remission and *boy did I feel it*. I had trouble sleeping, felt heavily fatigued, brain fogged and had muscle aches.

I went back to the functional medicine practitioner I had worked with before, for support in implementing the lifestyle factors I'd done previously and within three months, my Hashimoto's was back in remission and levels stabilised again. It is recommended to check your thyroid levels around 6 weeks after giving birth, 8 weeks after that and, if they have stayed stable and you feel well, twice yearly going forward.

When I received the news that my Hashimoto's was no longer in remission, was I surprised? No. Was I upset? Also no. Let me tell you why… Living with a health condition is rarely a smooth journey in the way that there will be times that it is under better control and times when it flares up again and this is especially true with a hormonal health condition, as there are so many factors that can affect it. My antibodies had only risen slightly, just over the normal range, but they had still risen and I was OK about that. Life is forever changing. My Hashimoto's was never going to be in remission forever and I knew this. There are so many reasons why Hashimoto's can flare back up again and antibodies rise. I expected pregnancy to do it, but it didn't. I expected it to flare up after giving birth, yet it surprised me by staying in remission until, there I was, six months postpartum, and after speaking to my functional medicine practitioner, I was reassured that this was not unusual at all. Hashimoto's coming out of remission can be caused by sudden illness, pregnancy, giving birth, stress, grief or an infection. So, to me, this was just another bump, another turn, another junction on my thyroid journey. I expected them to go back down again when the timing was right for my body, and that's exactly what happened. I focused on my adrenal health, gut health, diet, sleep, exercise and more to get things back on track and in remission again.

For some, their levels may bounce around for longer and require more monitoring until it settles again. Pregnancy and childbirth are huge stressors for the body and this shouldn't be ignored. Many of us require closer than usual monitoring to recover and find a new 'normal' during the postpartum period and first year or so of parenting. However, by the year mark, your levels should hopefully be settled. You may be on a higher dose of thyroid medication than you were pre-pregnancy, but if you're still feeling unwell, check which tests you are having run, which should include the full thyroid panel as well as Ferritin, Vitamin D and B12 which can deplete from pregnancy and birth. Any hair loss, muscle aches and pains or fatigue should also be explored with these tests. Postpartum hair loss is a common experience, but if it goes on for longer than a few months, then low thyroid levels or Ferritin could be behind it.

Exploring adrenal health following pregnancy and birth can be useful too, since pregnancy is a stress on the body and some support here can be much needed. Some people also experience migraines and headaches as they recover from pregnancy and childbirth and their thyroid hormone levels settle. I found that migraines were most present when my breast milk was establishing and my sleep was most disrupted in the newborn stage.

Tiredness

As parents with hypothyroidism and Hashimoto's, we can find it tricky to pinpoint what 'normal new parent tired' is, and what 'thyroid tired' feels like. How do we know what level of tiredness is actually normal for a new parent? I personally found that it felt much different. I would describe thyroid tired as:

Walking through treacle in lead boots. A shower tiring you out so much that you have to rest afterwards. Randomly falling asleep around a friend's house (and feeling rude for doing so). Getting fourteen hours of sleep or four hours of sleep and feeling exactly the same after both.

At my worst with thyroid fatigue, I felt like a twenty-one-year-old in a ninety-one-year-old's body. My ability to keep up work, relationships and housework was diminished. Some people are even unable to work.

Now, parenting (especially in the early days) can be exhausting! It takes a lot of physical and mental energy. There are sleepless nights, early morning starts and demands placed on you that can feel hard to keep up with. In my personal experience, 'new parent tired' is the closest it gets to 'thyroid tired', but it's still slightly different. Thyroid fatigue affects brain function in a heavier way, often leading to brain fog, reduced cognitive ability and forgetfulness that has been compared to dementia. Thyroid fatigue can also feel like you have the flu, affecting your ability to move around the house or get simple tasks done. When you're tired with young children, you often run on knowing that you still have to feed them, look after them and keep them alive, before falling into bed at the end of the day and thinking "Phew, I'm tired!"

Unfortunately, thyroid fatigue can leave you without the ability to do simple tasks for yourself, let alone anyone else. Thyroid fatigue isn't something you can just 'push through' and I found that that was the difference.

I covered thyroid flare days in Chapter 4, but once you become a parent, the usual tips and advice of 'rest as much as you can', 'don't overexert yourself' and 'fuel yourself properly' become much harder to follow. Navigating flares as a parent can be tricky because, among other things, you may not find it easy to get all the rest you need in order to recover quickly. As a parent myself, my top suggestions for navigating flares in this season of life include eating well where you can, cancelling plans, reviewing supplements and pulling in support where possible. In terms of eating as well as you can, this isn't always easy when you feel unwell and you have children screaming at you, but you can keep it simple. I like to put away extra portions of food in the freezer, labelled, for tough health days. If I decide I'm going to order takeaway due to a flare, I'll often try to find 'healthier' options such as salads, broths, Thai or Vietnamese food, or other trendy 'healthy food takeaway' restaurants. You'd be surprised at the options around now. Of course, having a less healthy takeaway for one night is unlikely to do a huge amount of damage either, so weigh up any stress involved. I just wouldn't recommend making it a frequent staple.

I also avoid sugar, caffeine and alcohol on flare days because these tend to make me feel worse. I'll instead fill up my water bottle with water and sip all day long to remain hydrated. I will add in extra Vitamin C and Zinc for a day or two if I'm in a flare, in order to support my immune system and body overall.

I'll stay home wherever I can, cancel social plans and anything nonessential. Yes, my child still requires looking after but a lot of errands can wait another day when I am hopefully more recuperated. I prioritise the essentials only and go into 'survival mode' so as not to drain myself further. I'll swap out more intensive exercise for yoga, or just not exercise at all if my body isn't up to it (it's important not to push it during a flare). I look for ways my child and I can do lower energy activities and if they're young enough that they still nap, I will squeeze in a nap myself or go for a bath to help with muscle pain.

And then lastly, pull in support where you can. Not all of us are lucky to have friends and family close by. I have often struggled with feeling lonely and isolated on tough thyroid days. However, you may be able to ask a family member or friend whether they could watch your child for an hour while you rest in bed, bring you a meal, or take your children for a playdate out the house?

Our top priority should be recuperating on fatigued days, wherever possible, otherwise we risk the fatigue dragging on for longer. Making small changes in order to reserve as much energy for recuperating as possible can really help. I hope these suggestions have given you some ideas!

Being a parent of a small baby is hard enough, but it can be extra hard managing your health on top of adjusting to a new, tiny human being you're suddenly responsible for. In the early days postpartum, I would forget to take my thyroid medication every day, the same for supplements, I found it hard to eat as healthily as I used to with so much less time and energy, I would plan to get out for daily walks but felt exhausted running on such little sleep from his night wakes and I found babywearing tiring too, even though it worked brilliantly at getting my babies to sleep while keeping me hands-free. The usual things I would do to manage my thyroid health and keep on top of it before I became a parent suddenly felt much trickier to maintain after my first son was born. I also found that it was much easier to trigger a thyroid flare. Navigating this isn't easy but we eventually settle into a new rhythm. Reach out to and connect with other mums, especially ones who also have health conditions. Then learn what your new rhythm looks like for this season of life. It will likely involve saying "No" to more things, setting firmer boundaries and prioritising your health.

Postpartum Thyroiditis

A condition called Postpartum Thyroiditis can show up after birth for both those who have an existing thyroid condition and those who do not. It is where the thyroid gland becomes inflamed after pregnancy, and this happens to around 5-7% of women, usually within a few months of giving birth. Interestingly, it is a form of autoimmune disease. Postpartum Thyroiditis usually presents as a painless, small enlargement of the thyroid, and can cause either hyperthyroid or hypothyroid symptoms. This can also lead to postpartum depression because of its impact on thyroid function. There are potentially two phases to postpartum thyroiditis. The inflammation and release of thyroid hormones into the blood usually first causes symptoms of hyperthyroidism:

- Anxiety
- Increased sensitivity to heat
- Insomnia
- Irritability
- Rapid heartbeat or palpitations
- Tremor
- Unexplained weight loss

These usually occur within a few months of giving birth. It is important to confirm if it is postpartum thyroiditis or Graves' disease with testing.

As thyroid cells are continually attacked, signs and symptoms of hypothyroidism can develop:

- Lack of energy/fatigue/weakness
- Increased sensitivity to cold/cold hands and feet

- Constipation
- Dry skin
- Difficulty concentrating/brain fog/confusion
- Aches and pains
- Depression

Most women who experience postpartum thyroiditis return to normal thyroid function after about a year, however, around a third develop permanent hypothyroidism.[40] [41]

Hashimoto's and a permanently underactive thyroid can also develop from the triggering of pregnancy. Many people find they are diagnosed with these a few months after giving birth.

How To Support Your Thyroid Postpartum

Coming towards the end of pregnancy with my first child in 2020, I was often wondering what postpartum had in store for me. I knew the usual stuff to expect; sleep deprivation with a newborn, a messy house and to have much less time to myself, but what about my physical health? What would the hypothyroidism and Hashimoto's look like? This naturally led me on to thinking about what I could plan or prepare to do, to support my thyroid health postpartum.

I'd lived with my thyroid condition for at least five years by this point and was familiar with thyroid flares, my Hashimoto's being in remission (and also not), thyroid medication dosage adjustments every now and then, as well as other pieces of my health such as adrenal dysfunction, low vitamin levels and how poor diet or the wrong exercise could make my thyroid condition worse. I made a plan of the things I could do postpartum in order to support getting my physical health back on track as smoothly as possible and support my thyroid health so that it would impact my experience as a new parent as little as possible too.

Even before we knew that our baby's first two years of life would be under pandemic restrictions, we had planned to keep the first month very simple for us all. We had made it clear to friends and family that visits would be very limited for the first month and that mostly, we would be focusing on staying at home, getting me recuperated and all three of us bonded as a new family unit. I also wanted to focus on establishing breastfeeding (especially knowing how hypothyroidism can impact this) and have plenty of time uninterrupted to feed.

We lowered our expectations regarding a clean house (and keeping visitors to an absolute minimum meant we felt even less pressure about this, too), kept the need to cook to a minimum with batch cooked, frozen meals and dedicated our limited time and energy only to essential tasks.

During pregnancy, I kept on top of testing my vitamin levels every few months and adjusting any supplements I was taking in line with this, so as to make sure I wasn't taking anything I didn't need and could therefore be dangerous, but also in order to support my physical health by ensuring I was getting enough of key vitamins and minerals needed for pregnancy and my thyroid health. After pregnancy, I carried this on, testing my levels (Ferritin, Vitamin D, B12 etc.) a month after giving birth and altering my regimen based on the results. My doctor also advised that I carried on the prenatal vitamin I started during pregnancy, for as long as I was breastfeeding.

I had to frequently remind myself that I was not only a new parent trying to figure all of this new, life changing information out, but I was also a new parent juggling my own chronic health condition. I needed to give myself some grace and manage my own expectations, because it was very easy to feel as if I was 'failing' for not doing exactly what all the other new parents were able to keep up with.

Whilst pregnant, I kept in mind that I may benefit from the input of a functional medicine practitioner after pregnancy, for support with my adrenal health, sex hormones and overall health and wellbeing. I wanted to support my body by recovering as smoothly as possible so that I could enjoy this new chapter in my life without my health getting in the way too much.

It wasn't until I was around six months pregnant that I felt I needed the support of a functional medicine practitioner, however. They were a great help. I also continued to see an NHS Midwife until I was a few weeks postpartum (visits happened at home), until they decided they were no longer needed. They would check over the baby and myself, performing mental health questionnaires and checks on my stitches. I had a very small, simple tear with my first birth, and did not tear with my second. Tears in pregnancy are common and usually heal fine with plenty of rest.

During pregnancy, my exercise routine had changed a lot. After birth, I focused solely on walking for the first four or five months, going very slowly and gradually increasing how long I would walk for as my body allowed and felt comfortable with. Eventually, I introduced yoga and swimming again, as well as aerobic workouts (I love dance cardio classes!), strength training and more intense exercise, but only as my body felt comfortable doing so. Over-exercising is a quick way to send your health plummeting with thyroid disease, so we really do have to be mindful.

Drinking bone broth each evening supported my gut health, adrenals and overall mission to holistically manage my health after pregnancy and childbirth, as well as breastfeeding.

What can we do about sleep? Prioritising sleep is definitely easier said than done with a new baby! Their sleep patterns (if they even have them) can be erratic at best, but in those first few months especially, I made sure to head to bed for the evening fairly early, anticipating that I'd be woken up a lot throughout the night. During the day, I found a balance in going out for an hour or two at most during the morning or afternoon, but not both, otherwise I'd be putting myself in thyroid flare territory. I also needed time at home.

I tried to avoid comparing myself to other mums (perhaps without chronic illnesses) who seemed to be able to do a lot more running around with their babies than me, and instead enjoyed soaking up days in the garden with my son or short walks over being out for long periods of time, which would deplete my restricted energy reserves even more so. (Refer back to the spoon theory in Chapter 3!)

As soon as my little one started to show signs of napping at the same sort of times each day and being able to go to sleep without much help from me (around the 3-4 month mark), I also prioritised being home for his nap times and bedtime, so that I could have a real rest for an hour or two. If you're always on the move while they nap, for example, pushing the pushchair / stroller or driving in the car, you're not making the most of the time you're not needed by them.

A note on independent sleep in babies: Some parents may consider gentle sleep training or creating predictable sleep routines for their baby, in order to increase the chances of better sleep for not only their child but also themselves, and therefore have more energy. Once my baby was sleeping more predictably, my thyroid condition and overall health was much better managed and stable.

Not a fan of the old school 'cry it out' methods, we sought the help of a baby sleep consultant to help us apply gentle sleep training methods which involved staying with the baby and providing comfort, slowly using less as he showed he needed it less. Sleep training is always controversial, but for me personally, I needed to be getting better sleep so that I could look after my children safely and be in better mental and physical health for them.

On a last note, I wanted to include a reminder that the general advice is to abstain from sex or strenuous activity for at least 6 weeks post-birth. Some people will need longer, so listen to your body and your doctor. The wound on the inside of your body (and possibly outside, if you had a C-Section) takes a lot more time to heal than people often realise.

Postpartum Weight Loss

We often feel the pressure to lose any extra weight after giving birth. I could say a lot about this, but I'll just say: I don't understand how we can go from celebrating a woman's body for growing, nurturing and birthing a whole human life, to berating her body to shrink back down and look as if it never did any of those things as soon as the baby is out. It's bananas.

Although it may be tempting to jump into a new weight loss plan as soon as possible, I would urge you to focus more on giving your body good nutrition instead. Doing so will yield results in your breastmilk production as well as your energy and also promote good thyroid health and stability in feeling well.

Think of your extra weight as an energy store for your baby and you in this postpartum stage, especially if you are breastfeeding, which causes you to burn more calories. Even if you are not breastfeeding, your body still requires nutrient dense food to replenish vitamin and mineral stores as well as heal from pregnancy and birth.

Our bodies usually settle to where they are happy, losing any excess weight, with optimised thyroid hormone levels, a balanced diet and regular exercise. I often hear the phrase "9 months on, 9 months off", implying that it takes 9 months to lose extra weight after birth, however, many women find it's more like 12-18 months. Your body will be individual. I encourage you to think about adopting a healthy *lifestyle* and focusing on how you *feel* over your weight alone. Your child wants you to be a present, mentally resilient parent, which should be a priority.

Pelvic Floor

If your pelvic floor muscles are weakened following pregnancy and birth, you may find that you leak urine, especially when you jump, cough or sneeze. This is really common, however, pelvic floor exercises can help to strengthen the pelvic floor muscles again. There are many apps and videos online talking you through these exercises. I personally loved the NHS app which would remind me at three points during the day to do my pelvic floor exercises. Speak to a healthcare professional if you are leaking urine (or stools) following birth.

End of Chapter Checklist:

- [ ] I have noted down who is in my support network for this new stage of life.
- [ ] I have had my thyroid levels checked 4-6 weeks after birth.
- [ ] I am having my thyroid levels checked every 2 months after birth until they are stable and optimal.
- [ ] I am having my thyroid levels checked twice a year once they are optimised and stable.
- [ ] I have considered whether I'd benefit from postpartum support by practitioners mentioned in Chapter 6. E.g. a Functional Medicine Practitioner, for holistic lifestyle support.
- [ ] I have had key nutrient levels checked; Ferritin, Vitamin D, B12 etc.
- [ ] Any postpartum hair loss has stopped within 3 months of starting. If not, thyroid and nutrient levels have been checked.
- [ ] I am utilising The Spoon Theory (Chapter 3) to find balance in my energy usage.
- [ ] I am managing flares with the tips mentioned in this chapter as well as Chapter 4.
- [ ] I am remembering to take any medications and supplements every day (set reminders if needs be!)
- [ ] I have considered postpartum thyroiditis / I have ruled it out.
- [ ] I am keeping the first few months simple, with limited house visits and a focus on bonding as a family and establishing feeding, the starts of new routines and recovery.
- [ ] I am still taking my prenatal (if breastfeeding).

- I am going slowly with reintroducing exercise following birth. I am listening to my body.
- I am drinking bone broth.
- I am prioritising sleep where I can - going to bed early, utilising naps, considering gentle sleep training (once baby is 3 months or older), and establishing some basic routines for naps and bedtime.
- I am abstaining from sex and other strenuous activity until I am 6 weeks postpartum / have been given the all clear by a doctor.
- I am doing pelvic floor exercises and discussing any leakages with a healthcare professional.
- I am focusing on nutrition and less so on weight loss.

Chapter 10: Postpartum Mental Health

Some postnatal depression cases are due to low thyroid function. This is a fact. Thyroid hormone is important for mental health, which can mean that depression, anxiety, mood swings and more can present with thyroid hormone levels which are too high or too low. The presence of thyroid antibodies can also impact mental health.

As well as obvious signs of your mental health being impacted, such as low moods, anxious thoughts and mood swings, other signs include not enjoying your baby / parenthood, feeling overwhelmed and having thoughts of harming yourself or your baby. Please seek support as soon as possible if you experience any of these.

Many of us experience tricky mental health periods after pregnancy and childbirth, so if this is you, please know that you are not alone. I had my first child during the 2020 pandemic, which definitely contributed to my diagnosis of postnatal depression.

I also want to make something very clear: antidepressants, anti-anxiety medication and more, can be a great help to many people struggling with their mental health, and it is important that we do not feed the stigma that taking these is 'wrong'.

I am not against medication for mental health, I am for making an informed decision, which means making sure those who are thyroid patients, perhaps also postpartum and experiencing mental health conditions, know that addressing their endocrine health fully may well resolve their mental health complaints and they may not need these additional medications.

In fact, I feel that thyroid screening should become mandatory during all pregnancies and postpartum and should be standard for anyone experiencing mental health struggles.

Thyroid hormone T3 has an important role in the health and optimal functioning of your brain, including: your cognitive function, ability to concentrate, mood, memory and attention span and emotions and ability to cope with life's stresses. T3 interacts with brain receptors and makes the brain more sensitive to chemicals such as Serotonin and Norepinephrine, which affects your alertness, memory, mood and emotions.

If you have had your thyroid levels checked and been told they're fine, please make sure they are in fact optimal (explained in Chapter 3), which can make a lot of difference, as well as that the full thyroid panel is being checked.

This includes:

- TSH
- Free T3
- Free T4
- Thyroid Peroxidase Antibodies
- Thyroglobulin Antibodies

Ensure you are taking your thyroid medication every single day, utilising reminders on your phone if required and not skipping doses. This has to be a priority to keep you in good health as a new parent. It may be that a new type of thyroid medication will be needed after pregnancy, as I found. My body's needs changed and I had to be open to this and find what would make me feel good and optimise my levels again. Chapter 3 covers different thyroid medication options.

If thyroid antibodies are high, signalling Hashimoto's, then lowering these can really help. My antibodies were high when I was 6 months postpartum, signalling that Hashimoto's came out of remission for me (this is common). By working to reduce these back down again and get it under remission once more, it went a long way in improving my mental and physical health. Chapter 3 covers strategies for this.

The same goes for levels of B12, Vitamin D and Ferritin following birth, which can be depleted due to the demands of pregnancy and childbirth, and thus contribute to poor mental health, brain fog, fatigue and more.

Adrenal dysfunction could also be causing or contributing to poor mental health. I've covered what adrenal dysfunction is in Chapter 3. Adrenal dysfunction can be common among thyroid patients, which may result in cell receptors failing to properly receive T3 from the blood, as well as make you feel as if you're constantly in stressed-out mode. Once adrenal dysfunction is addressed or when you are starting to recover from it, you may see your symptoms easing. It is then important to maintain good adrenal health going forward.

Prioritising sleep and recuperation where you can (I know firsthand that this isn't always easy - see the previous chapter for more on this), is also important for your mental wellbeing. Get extra sleep whenever you can if you feel you need it. Is someone visiting for a few hours and could watch the baby while you get a nap in? Or use that time for self-care, like a hot shower and a chance to brush your teeth. Self-care is important for mental health and isn't all bubble baths and spa days. It's the simple stuff too.

Struggles with mental health can have a biological cause, but also a situational one. Anxiety and depression can be driven by how you feel that your thyroid condition affects your ability to parent e.g. having low stamina, low energy, thyroid flares, aches, pains and more. You may feel frustrated if your thyroid condition 'gets in the way' of enjoying the early days of parenting as much as you thought you would. I know I did. Pregnancy can also cause changes in appearance, from weight gain to acne and hair loss. These changes can be upsetting and lead to low self-esteem or depression. Seeking support for these from a health professional and understanding that they will likely resolve with more time, helps. Please be kind to yourself.

Entering parenthood is a huge shift in our lives. I didn't feel as if I had the swing of things until my firstborn was at least six months old, and even then, I was still exhausted all the time and my thyroid health wasn't great.

By the time he was 18-months old, my health had been really stable for quite some time and we'd found a rhythm which worked for us and perhaps even more importantly, my health. This included finding the balance of how many hours a day I would be out of the house for, whether I saved my energy for the morning or afternoon, finding the time and energy to cook nutritious meals again and my little one finally sleeping through the night which meant I was also better rested.

Find your tribe with this new stage of life. Others navigating parenthood without pretending it is all rainbows and unicorns. I found there to be a bit of a toxic culture around new parents needing to love their new lives, love everything about being a parent and never complain, especially if it was a long journey to have that baby. *Oh no, you shouldn't complain.*

But this is so unhealthy and unhelpful. Find your tribe, perhaps at baby clubs, at the park or in online support groups. Those who want to share the cute photos and celebrate milestones as well as listen to and share in the harder experiences. Social media would have you believe that parenthood comes easily to everyone, but it really does not. My firstborn was very colicky (we didn't find out until he was a few months old that he had a dairy intolerance, which he was ingesting through my breastmilk and he also never latched properly which caused other issues), and when I say he screamed from around 8am to Midnight without stopping, not even to sleep or have a proper feed, I mean it. He was a really unhappy newborn and I wasn't a happy new mother. I struggled to find anyone to talk to about it. All the other new parents in my WhatsApp groups were glowing with pride and sharing cute photos, which I couldn't do, as I rarely took any photos of my baby due to him crying all day. Why would I take photos or videos of that?

I eventually bonded with a few other new mums who I could confide in about this, while also helping to uplift each other and share the good bits, too. Those friendships have become my closest friends even to this day. My eldest son grew out of the colicky stage by the time he was 4 months old and we solved the dairy intolerance issue, and these days, has no issue with dairy whatsoever. It was such a small period of time in my life but the support my tribe gave me in that time means the world to me. Our lasting friendships are built on that experience we went through together.

I have also found immense help in cognitive behavioural therapy, EMDR and counselling sessions with a therapist. Please seek out talking therapies and support if you are struggling.

End of Chapter Checklist:

- ☐ I have found my tribe.
- ☐ I have considered therapy.
- ☐ I have checked the full thyroid panel, including antibodies.
- ☐ I have considered if I need support for Hashimoto's.
- ☐ I have considered if I'd benefit from a different type of thyroid medication.
- ☐ I have tested key nutrient levels, Ferritin, Vitamin D, B12.
- ☐ I have considered my adrenal health.
- ☐ I have considered whether antidepressants etc. would be helpful (and checked if they are OK alongside breastfeeding - if applicable).
- ☐ I am ensuring that I take my thyroid medication every day.
- ☐ I am prioritising sleeping and resting where I can.
- ☐ I am making time for self-care, no matter how small.
- ☐ I am limiting my social media time, especially around anything depicting the 'perfect image of parenthood'.

Chapter 11: Breastfeeding With Hypothyroidism

I was super keen to breastfeed when I was pregnant with my first child, absorbing all and any information I could on it so as to give us the best chance. Breastfeeding your child gives them a great start in life, boosts their immune system and gut health. As someone who has health conditions, I wanted to do what I could to at least reduce the chances of my children suffering from health issues themselves, so choosing to breastfeed them was a top priority for me personally.

Does that mean that formula feeding your child is a terrible idea? Oh god no, a terrible idea would be the child being fed nothing at all or something completely inappropriate like a big bowl of pasta as soon as they're out of the womb! A fed and happy child with a happy parent is most important, so as you read this chapter, I want you to keep in mind that if you do not wish to breastfeed, or do but it doesn't work out for whatever reason, then you are still doing a great job for you and your family. How they are fed is such a small part of being a parent, and while, yes, being breastfed is linked with lower rates of infections, asthma, obesity, diabetes and SIDS, again, this is only one part of the puzzle. Genetics, other external environmental factors and more also factor into these.

Breastfeeding was not as easy as I had hoped for with my children, although I did 'push on' for a lot longer than I probably should have, given how severely it impacted both my mental and physical health. With my first baby, I had a persistent abscess in my right breast from when my milk came in until I stopped breastfeeding him. You read that right. I had a constant, large, painful infection for months on end but continued on, even though months of antibiotics did not ever fully resolve it, nor did *weekly* sessions of having the ridiculous amounts of pus drained out of my breast with a needle. The cause was my baby being unable to correctly and sufficiently latch, despite seeing countless breastfeeding and lactation experts. As a result, his little stomach was never full and he cried almost constantly (also due to the dairy intolerance mentioned in the last chapter). I was constantly physically unwell from this persistent infection. When he was a few months old, I realised that I couldn't continue to breastfeed. I was drained. We eventually moved to a non-dairy formula and it was the right decision for us. My infection resolved within a week of stopping breastfeeding and I could stop the antibiotics which were disrupting my gut. I was *physically and mentally* so much better for this decision and he was finally out of pain and experiencing a full stomach too. I didn't find it easy to call it quits. I cried about the loss of a specific bond I felt while breastfeeding.

My second child also had breastmilk for a little time before moving on to being exclusively formula fed. I combi-fed breastmilk and formula from the start and then eventually moved to formula only. I carried a lot of trauma from my first experience of breastfeeding and I couldn't go there again. My body felt destroyed by it. I was also carrying a lot of heartbreak and guilt for it not working out when I was so set on it.

Women have many reasons why breastfeeding may not work out for them. Both of my children are so far in great health and you wouldn't know if they had been breastfed for one day, one year or three years just by looking at them and their medical history. Do I know what their health will look like in the future? Of course not, but I made the best decisions

I could with the information and circumstances I had at the time and I regret nothing. This is parenting, ladies and gentlemen! This is what we do. We make the best decision based on what we have and we hope for the best.

So, does hypothyroidism prevent us from being able to breastfeed? For most people, thankfully not. However, it can come down to how well managed your thyroid condition is. This chapter will answer the most common questions I receive around breastfeeding with hypothyroidism.

In terms of my personal experiences, hypothyroidism itself did not impact my ability to produce milk and breastfeed. My struggles with breastfeeding were not thyroid related. In fact, I produced plenty of colostrum and milk, perhaps too much, which is why I was so prone to mastitis and abscesses. I was on Armour Thyroid when my first child was breastfeeding and Armour Thyroid and Levothyroxine together with my second.

Is It Safe for Someone with Thyroid Disease to Breastfeed?

I am often asked whether our thyroid medication for hypothyroidism (Levothyroxine, Armour Thyroid, Liothyronine etc.) is safe to take while breastfeeding and the answer is yes. In fact, it's crucial for our health as well as milk production. Your thyroid medication is crucial in your body being able to produce enough milk.

Will My Thyroid Medication Pass to The Baby?

When you're on the right amount of thyroid medication (not overmedicated) it only crosses into breast milk in minute amounts and has no adverse effects on the child.

Overmedication or hyperthyroidism is different, though. Taking more thyroid medication than your body needs can lead to it being passed on to the baby in larger amounts, so keep on top of regular blood tests and keep levels optimised and within range. Being overtreated for your hypothyroidism isn't a great idea and can also negatively affect milk supply.

Thyroid hormone levels swinging up and down may occur for a few months following delivery of your child, as your body and hormones settle. Bear with it and work with your doctor.

How Can Hypothyroidism Affect Milk Supply?

The hormone prolactin is responsible for the production of breastmilk and is stimulated by TRH (thyrotropin-releasing hormone) which in turn stimulates the production of TSH. If TRH is low (which is often seen in those with low thyroid hormone levels – untreated or undertreated hypothyroidism) prolactin may also be low which can lead to low breastmilk production. Therefore, it is not uncommon for people with hypothyroidism to have issues with breastmilk production, but we can overcome and prevent it by maintaining optimal thyroid hormone levels throughout pregnancy and postpartum. Having your TSH, Free T3 and Free T4 levels checked soon after birth and regularly thereafter and optimising them is therefore crucial for good milk supply.

Signs you may have a milk supply issue include:

- Your baby is losing weight or gaining weight slower than is expected.
- A lack of wet and dirty nappies.
- Your baby is fussing at the breast and still hungry after a long feed.

You should speak to your paediatrician, midwife, family doctor, or a breastfeeding and lactation specialist regarding any concerns around these.

To support you with breastfeeding, a breastfeeding and lactation consultant can be invaluable as they will check the baby's latch, sucking strength, check for a tongue tie, and offer guidance with pumping and supplements to stimulate milk supply.

A book I have found invaluable on breastfeeding is *The Positive Breastfeeding Book by Amy Brown*, which covers the many ways in which we can support our breastfeeding journey as best as possible, and talks about tongue ties, latch, pumping, supplements etc. for encouraging a well-fed baby. The La Leche League website also has lots of helpful information.

On another note, if you are trying to lose weight in this postpartum period, by cutting calories, then this can impact your breastmilk supply too. A breastfeeding woman needs around 500-700 more calories every day, and if you don't have enough, your breastmilk supply can be compromised. See Chapter 9 for more information.

Will Breastfeeding Affect My Thyroid Levels?

Will breastfeeding affect thyroid hormone levels and create a need for more thyroid hormone replacement medication and a dosage increase? The answer is: it depends on your body. There is anecdotal evidence to say that some people require an increase in thyroid medication when they start breastfeeding, but this is also taking place directly after pregnancy and birth. Therefore, how can we be sure that it is the demand for breastmilk increasing the need for an increase in thyroid medication? Many find that they simply require a higher dosage of their thyroid medication after pregnancy anyway.

Conclusion

So yes, your thyroid hormone replacement medication is a crucial component of producing enough milk, as is the need for regular and comprehensive thyroid testing. It is not unusual to see milk supply issues in new parents with hypothyroidism, but this is often resolved with correct management of the thyroid condition and support from breastfeeding specialists.

Breastfeeding is often depicted as something that comes easily and naturally to mother and baby, but the truth is, it's often a skill that both parties need to learn and practise. Many of us set out with the best of intentions to breastfeed and I was devastated when I had to call it quits with my first child. I wasn't ready to. Please remain kind to yourself and keep in mind that you should do whatever works for you, your family, your mental health, wellbeing and preferences.

Many women do not feel comfortable breastfeeding for a variety of reasons, whether due to past trauma, abuse, it feeling painful and uncomfortable or feeling the urge to have their body back after all the demands of pregnancy. Many do not enjoy feeling as if they are the only person who can feed the baby. Many do not like wearing breastfeeding bras, breast pads, leaking milk and smelling of breastmilk. It's not easy to give up so much of your body for so long. Others may have physical challenges that prevent the ability to breastfeed, such as not having breasts due to a mastectomy or having transitioned / being in the process of, or having inverted nipples, or recurrent mastitis and abscesses.

Some choose to breastfeed. Some choose to pump and bottle feed their breastmilk. Some wish to solely formula feed. Others may do a mixture. There is also the option to locate donated breastmilk. There is no *one* correct way to feed your baby.

Please be mindful of online spaces who are very passionate about this topic. As a new mother who was finding breastfeeding extremely difficult, painful and very detrimental to my physical and mental health (due to the abscess, weekly hospital draining procedures and constant antibiotics), I felt I had no option but to keep on going due to the online push for pro-breastfeeding. And I get it, it provides a lot of benefits if you *can* give your child breastmilk. I knew all of this and as someone with a thyroid condition and well aware of all the benefits breastmilk gives to a child's health, I perhaps was *too* focused on this alone. In the end, I needed to accept that it just wasn't working and I wasn't a bad parent for closing that chapter. I really did do my best.

End of Chapter Checklist:

- ☐ My thyroid levels are optimised.
- ☐ I have sought the help of a breastfeeding / lactation specialist if I need some support.
- ☐ My baby has been checked for a tongue tie and correct latch.
- ☐ I have considered if pumping would be useful.
- ☐ I have explored supplements for milk supply, e.g. fennel, fenugreek (run past a pharmacist)
- ☐ My baby is gaining weight as expected.
- ☐ My baby has plenty of wet and dirty nappies.
- ☐ My baby seems content while feeding and full and happy afterwards.

Chapter 12: Parenting With Hypothyroidism

I wanted to start this chapter with an excerpt from my second book *"You, Me and Hypothyroidism: When Someone You Love Has Hypothyroidism"*. This book talks to our friends and family about the impacts of thyroid disease on various aspects of our lives.

"Raising a family when you have hypothyroidism can understandably bring with it added things to juggle. Just like during pregnancy, predicting someone's thyroid health when they have the added task of everything that comes with parenthood can become tricky. We all have an idea of who we want to be as parents, so imagine the guilt, regret and feelings of failure your loved one may feel when they feel as if they're coming up short due to their health condition leaving them with less energy, less time and less of the stuff they want to do in order to be a 'perfect parent'.

Of course, you probably feel that they are in fact doing enough, but they may not be feeling that way themselves. As you've probably gathered by now, thyroid patients are often known to push themselves each and every day to keep on going, keep on raising their families with love and kindness despite their own body fighting against them. Many parents with hypothyroidism are even more exhausted, even more stressed and struggle even more so mentally, as well as physically, than other parents.

On thyroid flare up days, pulling the laundry out of the washing machine can be exhausting, showering can use up all their energy and cooking the family a nutritious meal might not be an option if they're so fatigued and in pain that they're struggling to stand for long.

It's hard to say for any of us, whether our health will A) bounce back after beginning parenthood B) take a while and a mixture of different health practitioners to iron it back out or C) never truly be the same… If you embark on the journey of raising a family together, it may be that at times you need to remind them to check in with their doctor to have their thyroid levels checked and medication reviewed, as juggling their own medications, medical appointments and check-ups for themselves, let alone all the ones for your child or children too, can become overwhelming. And there's a good chance they'll be putting the kids first almost all the time.

When you have children, being realistic about both of your responsibilities as parents, such as whether you need to pull in help from a wider circle of support, is crucial… Support groups for parents in the community can be a lifeline. Regular meetups at parks, libraries, and more can provide great friendship, reassurance and support to both mothers and fathers. It may be that you utilise this form of support too, as it is possible that you may be able to connect with other parents that have a chronically ill other half."

On a thyroid flare day it can feel impossible to parent. I know because I've been there too. I know I felt like I was going from finally feeling like I was in a rhythm of managing my thyroid condition well to being turned upside down again once I became a parent! How on Earth do I do all that while also raising a human being (and wanting to do a good job of that too)? I hope this chapter gives you the confidence to go into parenting with a thyroid condition to manage as well.

Prioritise Fuelling Yourself

When you're pregnant, or even before then if you're able to, get into the habit of freezing extra portions of food that can be used for quick and nutritious meal options in the early postpartum days and beyond. If you're able to pull a meal from the freezer and have something ready to eat in just a few minutes, you'll be fuelled to tackle those colicky newborn days, the rushed-off-your-feet with a non-stop toddler days and any flare days that pop up. Staying well-fuelled with good food choices (think lots of protein, some carbs and a rainbow of veggies) will make parenting so much easier, I promise you. I'm pretty sure that if I didn't do this in the early days, then I'd have been eating takeaways and reaching for foods that were void of much nutrition a whole lot more during the first year or two of parenthood, and doing this makes me feel even more tired and sluggish and flares up my thyroid symptoms. Now my children are a little older (they're four and two as I write this book), I get them involved in the cooking. They like to watch me chop vegetables (and also give it a go where it's safe) and we sing as we stir pots. Invest in a 'learning tower' for your child so they can safely join you at the kitchen counter and you'll find cooking with them a lot smoother.

Let's not forget about hydration. The best way to stay hydrated is to carry a water bottle with you all day, even at home. Look for BPA and BPS-free water bottles that won't interfere further with your hormonal health. I fill up my water bottle (or a large drinking glass) first thing in the morning and sip it all day long. Every time I see the water bottle sitting on the sofa, table or in the pushchair when out and about, I sip. If I don't keep on top of staying hydrated, I soon become fatigued, cranky and develop a headache. Feeling that way certainly doesn't help with caring for a little one! Being dehydrated is also a quick way to get yourself constipated, which is another dreaded hypothyroid symptom.

Dealing With Disrupted Sleep

If I don't make sure I'm in bed by 10pm, I feel awful the next day. When you have a little person waking you up in the night and then needing you on demand all day, do whatever you can to get as much sleep at night as possible.

Boosting Your Mornings

Early morning starts are often another way in which our thyroid condition can be impacted. When my second child went through a year-long phase of starting the day at 5:30am I found it so rough on the management of my thyroid condition. I experienced more flare days (lack of sleep is the biggest cause of those for me), more headaches and migraines, and as well as the obvious extra fatigue, brain fog would go through the roof too.

I'm hoping you're not having as early a start as I did, but just in case you are, or if whatever time your little one is starting the day feels just too early, I hope the following tips help.

1. Stick to a Bedtime Routine

To have energy in the morning, one of the best things we can do is ensure we get to bed at a reasonable time every night, factoring in how often your little one wakes up. For example, a newborn wakes frequently during the night, so you will feel better if you head to bed early to factor in all the wake-ups. Once they start sleeping through the night, you likely won't need to head to bed as early but depending on what time they start the day, you may need to alter your own bedtime. For example, when I only had my first child, who never woke up before 7am and slept through the night, I could go to bed at 11pm and wake at 7am feeling rested. My second child has always been more likely to wake up during the night and also start the day earlier, so I need an earlier bedtime myself since having him, usually heading to bed at 10pm. Figure out a realistic time to be in bed for you. It can be tempting to stay up later to enjoy some child-free time, but if you do, you may regret it the next day if thyroid fatigue is rife.

For the last hour or two before bed, step away from screens (TV, phone, laptop), change any bright lights to warmer lamps and find activities that help you to wind down. These can include meditation, reading a book or taking a soothing bath (with Epsom Salts) or shower. Using electronics too late in the evening can interfere with your production of melatonin, the 'sleep hormone'.

2. Take Your Thyroid Medication

Please make sure you're taking your thyroid medication every day. Missing doses of your thyroid medication can lead to you feeling rather unwell and fatigued, especially in the mornings.

3. Swap Mindless Scrolling for Something Engaging

What you're exposed to when you wake up impacts your first thoughts and feelings of the day. Instead of reaching straight for your phone and scrolling mindlessly, perhaps seeing some negative content upon waking, put some uplifting music on and ban the news and social media for the first hour of your day. I switch it up and listen to music or an uplifting podcast depending on my mood. Music can be really powerful, especially your favourite feel-good songs, so create a playlist of them and make them part of your morning routine. Dancing with my children is one of my favourite mood-boosting activities!

4. Fuel Your Body

Breakfast is the most important meal of the day. Having a health condition that affects energy levels, it is crucial that we give our bodies the best start to the day possible, with a substantial, energy-boosting breakfast. Research has shown that having Hashimoto's puts us at an increased risk of blood sugar imbalances or glycaemic impairments and this then places extra stress on our adrenals, which isn't helpful.[42]

The best options for a blood sugar balancing breakfast revolve around protein, which can include: eggs, meat, cheese, quinoa and nuts. Switching sugary cereal for porridge topped with nut butter, or jam on toast for chicken sausages and toast, I've noticed this small change makes a big difference in how I feel in the morning.

5. Get Yourself Moving, Even a Little Bit

I'm not saying you have to go for a run first thing in the morning, but some gentle exercise to help warm up your body and get blood pumping can be a good way to start your day. Gentle stretches, such as yoga, can be done in just a few minutes and give your body a gentle wake up to the day. YouTube provides free videos and tutorials and you can do them beside your bed if needs be!

Now, if running in the morning *is* your thing, check-out those 'running pushchairs' for babies, and once your child is older, have them go for a run with you! My four-year-old son loves going for a run with his dad.

Making Time for Rest

I felt worn out by the time my first baby was six months old because I was trying to keep up with the other mums. They were taking their babies out and socialising every day. When I tried to do this too, my health suffered. I was SO tired. I figured out that my happy medium involved taking my baby out a few times a week and only for a few hours at most each time. Sometimes just an hour was long enough. If I did more than this, I soon brought on thyroid flares. On top of the sleep deprivation, going out and doing too much too often was a recipe for disaster when it came to managing my health. I also made Fridays a PJ Day for a while! During the first year of his life, my son and I would spend Fridays in our pyjamas, at home and with very little planned. This would allow me some time to recuperate a little before the weekend.

A lot of people also nap during the day when their little one does, or opt to go out in the morning, staying home in the afternoon or vice versa. I particularly love this balance and have alternated whether we get out for an hour in the morning and relax at home for the afternoon, or do it the other way round, depending on where we currently are and what works. I briefly felt a little anxious that I wasn't 'parenting right' by organising my day in this way, but then I remembered something that is often not at the forefront of my mind these days; I have a chronic illness. I'm a mum, yes, but I also have health conditions to keep in mind and other mums do not, and so they may be able to cope with being busier than I am.

Learning how to balance things so that I wasn't completely exhausted was a real learning curve and that included turning down invites to afternoon activities because we were out all morning.

It's OK to set boundaries as a parent with chronic illness. It's OK to not overcommit and feel as if you have to jam-pack your day. It's OK if you don't conform to this expectation that mums should be out all day and non-stop busy with their children. You do whatever works for you, your health and your family.

Also, when we have chronic health conditions and especially with thyroid issues, it's helpful to carry on reassessing our current needs and abilities over time. For some seasons of life, you may be able to tolerate more or higher intensity exercise, and for others: less.

A couple months postpartum, my husband and I agreed that he would start taking the baby out for an hour each Saturday morning so that I could have a bath, wash my hair, shave my legs and have some regular 'me time' which I could look forward to each week. It made a big difference in how I felt, mentally and physically. I also started prioritising time for other things that impact my overall health and wellbeing, such as reading books, gardening and baking. When my children would go for a nap (neither nap anymore sadly!), I would allow myself just fifteen minutes maximum for cleaning and 'boring adult jobs' and then would make myself sit and enjoy a book with a cup of tea for the remainder of their nap. If you frequently find yourself saying "I don't have time for X", try saying "I don't prioritise time for X" instead and see how that makes you feel. What steps can you take to change this?

I started small by making time for a bath each week and built it up from there. Nowadays, I attend my weekly dance cardio classes on a weekday evening again, the same goes for a yoga class, and I ensure I read at least a page or two of my book every day. I prioritise the things that make me 'me' because I know that it's important for my health and wellbeing as well as for my children to see a good example of someone maintaining hobbies, health, boundaries and more.

Can I Prevent a Thyroid Condition in My Child?

For so many of us, it was a long journey to the diagnosis of a thyroid condition and possibly an even longer one back to good health (if you're there yet). Getting on the right type and dosage of thyroid medication for you can take a while, as can finding a good thyroid literate doctor and implementing any lifestyle changes and other jigsaw puzzle pieces you need (such as supplements, gut health, diet and stress management). I personally didn't just struggle with my physical health, but my mental health was also hugely impacted by an undiagnosed and non-optimally treated thyroid condition for years and the thought of any future children having the same experience as I used to give me anxiety. Of course, no parent wants their child to suffer with something that could be more easily diagnosed and treated, so naturally, you may wonder whether there is a way to avoid your child developing a thyroid condition at all. Can we prevent this?

Let's start with the cause of hypothyroidism in most of us and what triggers that. In around 90% of us with hypothyroidism, we have the autoimmune disease Hashimoto's Thyroiditis to thank for it. As explained in Chapter 1, this autoimmune condition causes the thyroid gland to lose function as time goes on, therefore, for most of us, it is actually the triggering of Hashimoto's that we are talking about. How is this triggered? It is believed that those of us carrying the genetic makeup to develop Hashimoto's trigger the condition by switching it 'on'.

We know that there is a combination of genetics and environment at play for triggering a thyroid condition, and that there are often multiple triggers and contributors too.

The most common triggers are:

- Hormonal shifts (such as puberty, starting or stopping hormonal contraceptives, pregnancy, postpartum and the menopause)
- Big life stressors (such as bereavement, family dysfunction, abuse)
- Adrenal stress in the form of continued high cortisol levels for a long time (often associated with people who feel anxious for a lot of the day, burn the candle at both

ends and do not have time for rest, downtime or hobbies)
- Iodine deficiency or excess Iodine
- Other low nutrient levels, such as Vitamin D or Iron
- A blow to the immune system such as a severe illness or virus
- Gut issues / poor gut health

So now that we know what these are, we can just make sure that our children avoid them, right? It's unlikely to be that simple. While we may be able to avoid *some* possible triggers, there are others that we just cannot avoid entirely. Therefore, it is impossible to completely prevent our children from developing a thyroid condition if they have inherited the ability to do so from us.

For example, life is stressful. It just is. We can't prevent all terrible things from happening that may cause enough of a stress response that a thyroid condition such as Hashimoto's is triggered. We also cannot prevent our children from catching any illnesses, or prevent puberty. We can certainly look at the possible triggers and ask ourselves what we can do to reduce the chances of them triggering a thyroid condition. For example, we can create a focus on good nutrition, meaning that we eat everything in balance, focusing on whole foods wherever we can, to support good gut health and nutrient levels, reducing the risk of these becoming triggers.

Some thyroid sources will say that children should be eating gluten-free, dairy-free, soy-free and more to avoid triggering a thyroid issue, but there is a major lack of evidence to suggest this works or is really necessary. I'm very cautious about restricting children's diets because it may lead to nutritional deficiencies, as well as disordered eating behaviour that can be hard to undo later on. Obviously, if your child has food allergies, intolerances or sensitivities, then work with a professional to keep these properly managed.

In terms of looking after their adrenal health so as to limit the chances of this triggering a thyroid condition, we can look at instilling a respect for movement and exercise, finding what works for our bodies whilst also being mindful of over-exercising. Teaching healthy sleep habits (how to prioritise and value good sleep), that we need time for rest and hobbies and anything else that keeps our cortisol levels under control for most of the time can also be invaluable in our children. Cortisol is a very useful hormone and its presence is not an issue unless levels of it are excessively high for long periods of time, so we would want to avoid that. We can also aim to equip our children with the knowledge they need to process and deal with life's stressors, as well as the full range of emotions that we feel as humans. Processing our emotions healthily can teach us how to be much more resilient and well-balanced, with better mental health outcomes.

Books I have found helpful as a parent teaching this in my children include *Sometimes I Feel Sunny* by Gillian Shields, *My Body Sends a Signal* by Natalia Maguire, *I Feel Anxious* by Aleks Harrison, *Ruby's Worry* by Tom Percival and *The Growth Mindset Ninja* by Mary Nhin. All of these books focus on nurturing a child's emotional intelligence and resilience which can support healthier mental health and adrenal health throughout life.

If you are currently pregnant and wondering if there is anything you can do while pregnant to reduce the chances of your child having thyroid issues, then there is evidence that the mother maintaining adequate levels of thyroid hormone throughout pregnancy reduces the chances of a child being born with congenital hypothyroidism or health issues themselves. Therefore, regular blood testing (often every 4-6 weeks throughout) and suitable medication dosage adjustments can be very beneficial to the health of the child.

We may not be able to 100% prevent our children from developing thyroid issues like us, but these areas could go a way in reducing the chances or delay its onset. After all, since many cases are triggered by hormonal shifts in pregnancy, postpartum and menopause, these later causes are not entirely preventable, however, we can be mindful and make our children aware also. If Hashimoto's, Hypothyroidism or other thyroid conditions run in your family, you can be aware of any signs in your children and help them to be knowledgeable of the signs and symptoms too, so they do not go undiagnosed for long. We can have their thyroid levels tested as children and teenagers so we have a baseline of what is their 'normal', but also see any early warning signs of things changing.

I triggered Hashimoto's in my mid-teens by hammering a lot of triggers at once. I had two separate, severe strains of flu in the space of 18 months. I was also raised in a very dysfunctional, high-stress family environment and home. I did not sleep at all well, and had never learned how to deal or cope with stress and tricky emotions. My family dysfunction peaked in my teen years and thus, I triggered my thyroid issues. With my own children, I am focusing on good nutrition, teaching them to respect sleep and rest as well as finding exercise and movement they love and to speak about their feelings – the whole range of emotions – as well as find healthy ways to process them and build resilience. I protect them from the dysfunctional upbringing I had and try my best to parent in a way very different to what I experienced, but the kind of parenting and home life I needed as a child, which, had I received myself, I very likely would not have triggered a thyroid condition or perhaps it would have been triggered later on in life, giving me more time to enjoy life carefree. I also feel confident that should my children develop thyroid conditions, I will be their best advocate for testing, treatment and teaching them all I know so that it won't impact their life much at all.

My third book *Thyroid Superhero: A Kid's Guide to Understanding Their Grown-up's Hypothyroidism* teaches children about the signs and symptoms of hypothyroidism, as it covers how it impacts the adults in their life. It is also a great tool for raising awareness of the symptoms in your children.

End of Chapter Checklist:

- ☐ I am fuelling my body with nutritious food, especially in the morning.
- ☐ I am staying hydrated throughout the day.
- ☐ I am maximising how many hours of sleep I can get.
- ☐ I am carving out a bedtime routine for myself, prioritising time to wind down.
- ☐ I am taking my medications and supplements every day.
- ☐ I consume positive messaging in the morning, swapping social media or the news for audiobooks, music or podcasts.
- ☐ I exercise regularly.
- ☐ I am managing my spoons and expectations of everything I have to juggle as a parent with chronic illness.
- ☐ I am carving out time for self-care (such as my Saturday morning bath example).

RACHEL HILL

Extra Resources

A Letter To My 2020 Baby…

What a year it has been. It started with excitement to meet you and then, before not too long, we finally met. One final push, you took your first breath, I scooped you up in my arms and exclaimed "I know you!"

You wrapped your tiny hand around my finger and we gazed into each other's eyes.

Existing in our little bubble, we paid little attention to what was going on outside, as we focused on learning how to breastfeed, read your cries, soothe you to sleep and be a family of three.

Before long, the world was plunged into a strange existence. At just a couple of weeks old, just as we were starting to brave leaving the house, the country (and most the world) was told to stay in their homes for months on end. The pandemic hit when I was a brand new parent.

In many ways, 2020 has been a chaotic, confusing, scary mess.

Yes, the pandemic has been hard, but those first few months we had with you, completely alone and in desperate need of others, made it a thousand times harder. Your painful cries did not go unheard as we struggled to calm them. You cried harder and harder, we knew something was wrong, but without the ability to see a medical professional, it took a long time to resolve. A dairy intolerance was finally diagnosed.

Despite your mummy and daddy falling to pieces, you were the light in the darkness of these dark times. By focusing on you and you alone, it got us through. Parenting like this was not what we had planned, nor what we needed when I had a chronic health condition, let alone also navigating the breastfeeding challenges, my persistent breast infection and your milk intolerance.

Yes, it has been tough, but, my 2020 baby, I am so grateful that this year also brought us you. Your gurgles, your smiles, your first roll, your first day of crawling and your first "Mama". You are such a gift and light in what has been a somewhat dark and lonely year.

The first year of your life and my maternity leave is nothing like we expected or planned for – it's been lonelier and harder to navigate – but that's OK. I have you.

As we spend another long day together, just the two of us, I realise that your timing couldn't really have been any more perfect. ***You*** *couldn't have been any more perfect.*

Just as you grow day by day and week by week, I grow from the extra challenges this year has brought.

2020 has been hard, but you've made it easier to bear.

And I think we're starting to get the hang of this new normal.

Love, Mama x

***

I wanted to include this letter I wrote to my six-month-old son in 2020, to show just how far we have come. You've got this too.

Tests You May Need and Where to Order Them

Always work with a medical professional when evaluating and re-evaluating your thyroid hormone levels, keeping in mind your symptoms and overall health as well.

Places You Can Order Tests

Please note that any services included in this list are not necessarily endorsed or recommended by me. This list is kept up to date on my website, so know that you can check this online too, for any new testing companies I have become aware of.

In alphabetical order:

- **www.bloodtestslondon.com** - UK
- **Blue Horizon Blood Tests** - UK
- **DirectLabs** - USA
- **Genova Diagnostics** - International
- **i-Screen (App)** - Australia
- **LetsGetChecked** - UK, USA, Ireland
- **Medichecks** - UK
- **Medivere Diagnostics** - Germany
- **Monitor My Health** - UK
- **My Med Lab** - USA
- **NutriPATH** - USA, Canada, UK, South America, Switzerland, UAE, Asia, Australia, NZ
- **Ortho-Analytic** - Switzerland
- **Paloma Health** - USA

- **Private MD labs** – USA
- **www.privatebloodtests.co.uk** - UK
- **Smart Nutrition** - UK
- **Thriva** - UK
- **TrueHealthLabs** - UK, USA, Canada, Most of the world
- **ZRT Laboratory** - USA

List of Thyroid (And Related) Events

I thought a good addition to this book would be a list of events held around the world that recognise thyroid disease and raise awareness of it. Add these to your calendar if you wish to be reminded. I take part in these every year.

In month order:

Thyroid Awareness Month

Always held in January.

Autoimmune Disease Awareness Month

Always held in March.

International Women's Day

Always held on 8th March.

Hashimoto's and hypothyroidism are predominantly female health conditions and the issues around many women going undiagnosed or undertreated for so long has been called a 'feminist issue'. Using this annual awareness day can be great for urging other women to become more aware of thyroid disease so they're diagnosed sooner.

International Thyroid Awareness Week

Always held in May.

World Thyroid Day

Always held on 25th May.

World Head and Neck Cancer Day

This is held on the 27th of July each year. This is relevant due to Thyroid Cancer being located in the neck. Thyroid cancer often leads to hypothyroidism.

Thyroid Cancer Awareness Month

Always held in September. Again, many thyroid cancer survivors go on to be hypothyroidism patients.

Pregnancy and Infant Loss Awareness Month

Always held in October. Having a thyroid condition puts you at a higher risk for losing an unborn child.

World Mental Health Day

Always held on 10th October, we also know that mental health conditions often come hand in hand with thyroid disease.

Further Sources of Information

Thank you for reading this book. I really hope you have found it helpful on your journey to parenthood with a thyroid condition.

You can find more of my work, join my thyroid community and get in touch with me on:

- **My website**: theinvisiblehypothyroidism.com
- **My email newsletters**: https://theinvisiblehypothyroidism.substack.com/
- **Threads**: @theinvisiblehypothyroidism
- **Facebook**: Search 'The Invisible Hypothyroidism'
- **Instagram**: @theinvisiblehypothyroidism
- **Twitter**: @invisible_hypo
- **TikTok**: @invisiblehypothyroidism

As well as my website, social media platforms and newsletters, the below resources may also be helpful to you. They are not necessarily endorsed by me, and content may of course change with time, but they are worth exploring.

Please also consider leaving an online review of this book, so that other people can gauge if it will be a useful tool for them. Amazon, Goodreads etc. are great places to do this.

Books:

- **The Positive Birth Book** by Milli Hill
- **The Positive Breastfeeding Book: Everything you need to feed your baby with confidence** by Amy Brown

- **Mindful Hypnobirthing: Hypnosis and Mindfulness Techniques for a Calm and Confident Birth** by Sophie Fletcher
- **Healing Your Body Naturally After Childbirth** by Dr Jolene Brighten
- **The Pregnancy Encyclopedia** by Paula Amato and Dr Chandrima Biswas
- **What to Expect When You're Expecting** by Heidi Murkoff
- **Your Healthy Pregnancy with Thyroid Disease** by Dana Trentini and Mary Shomon
- **Beyond The Pill** by Dr Jolene Brighten
- **Hashimoto's Thyroiditis: Lifestyle Interventions for Finding and Treating the Root Cause** by Izabella Wentz PharmD
- **Hashimoto's Protocol** by Izabella Wentz, PharmD, FASCP
- **The Thyroid Hormone Breakthrough** by Mary J. Shomon
- **What You Must Know About Hashimoto's Disease** by Brittany Henderson MD
- **Thyroid Disease in a Nutshell** by Jules Chandler
- **Rethinking Hypothyroidism** by Antonio C. Bianco MD

Thyroid Cookbooks as Mentioned in Chapter 3:

- **The 30-Minute Thyroid Cookbook** by Emily Kyle MS, RDN, CDN, CLT and Rachel Hill
- **The Hormone Healing Cookbook** by Dr Alan Christianson

- **The Nourished Thyroid: A gluten-free and thyroid friendly cookbook for all lifestyles** by Nicole Morgan RDN LD CLT

Podcasts:

- The Goode Health Podcast
- Thyroid Healthy Bites Podcast
- Girls Gone Wellness Podcast
- Fempower Podcast
- Feel Better, Live More Podcast

Websites:

Dr Jolene Brighten

A women's health expert with thyroid disease herself. She covers fertility, birth control, hormonal conditions and more.

Hypothyroid Mom

Dana went through the traumatic experience of losing her unborn child when doctors failed to monitor her hypothyroidism correctly. She started blogging and advocating to change thyroid treatment and save more babies.

ITT – Improve Thyroid Treatment Campaign

Mission statement of the ITT:

- To press for improved diagnosis, testing & individualised treatment of thyroid disorders, for the benefit of all thyroid patients in the UK.
- To campaign for a range of treatment options and stop the removal of liothyronine (T3) by Clinical Commissioning Groups and Health Boards in the UK.
- To promote better understanding and education regarding the complexities of thyroid disease.
- To use members' reports of local or national difficulties to inform our campaign.

If you are looking for improved treatment and management of thyroid disease in the UK, and wish for other treatment options besides T4-only Levothyroxine to be available on the NHS, this is the group to get involved in.

Mary Shomon: Thyroid Patient Advocate

Thyroid patient advocate Mary Shomon has various books and website articles on thyroid disease, with many also covering fertility and pregnancy.

Thyroid Patient Advocacy

A UK charity, TPAUK is an independent organisation that works towards establishing better diagnosis and treatment of hypothyroidism.

The Thyroid Pharmacist, Izabella Wentz

Dr. Wentz is a well-respected expert in the thyroidsphere. She is a pharmacist who also developed Hashimoto's and through her own knowledge as a medical professional, has reversed her Hashimoto's and shares all this knowledge in her online content as well as her many books.

The Thyroid Trust

This UK thyroid charity is able to offer information and support on their Website, Social Media Channels and through their face to face patient voices and online cafe events, all as part of their mission to make things better for thyroid patients.

Thyroid Patients Canada

Thyroid Patients Canada is a nonprofit corporation registered with the Government of Canada. They promote health by providing individuals with thyroid disabilities with access to patient-led peer support communities and science-based public education, and by publicly advocating for improvements to thyroid health care policy and research.

Thyroid UK

Thyroid UK is a UK charity that works on improving the diagnosis and treatment of thyroid disease and are often at the front of campaigns.

Also by The Author

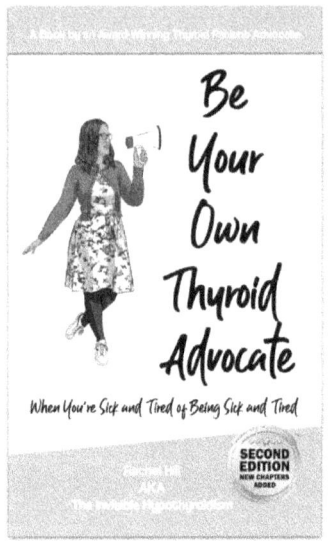
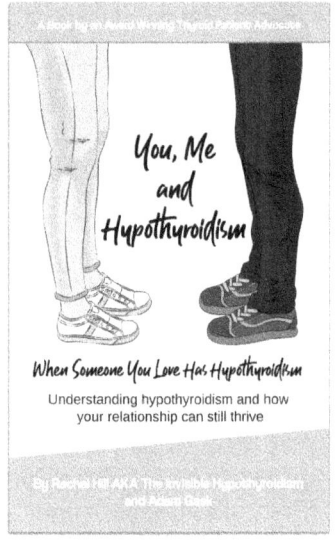

A complete and must-have resource for people with hypothyroidism.

The first resource for friends, family and other loved ones of thyroid patients.

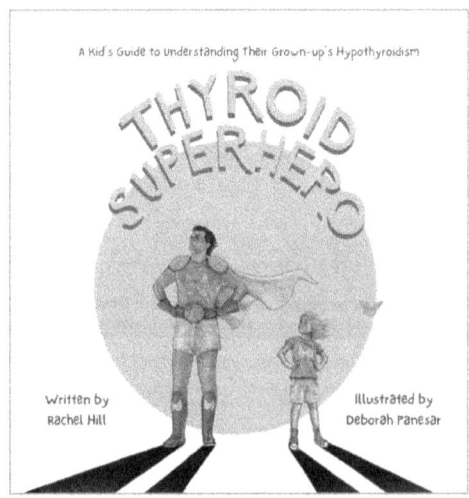

A children's book for understanding their grown-up's hypothyroidism.

Index

Adenomyosis, 56, 57, 62, 64
Adrenal, 11, 29, 49, 52, 55, 58, 59, 72, 73, 76, 77, 80, 82, 83, 104, 126, 167, 168, 173, 175, 176, 183, 200, 204, 206
Alcohol, 49, 66, 76, 79, 86, 106, 112, 115, 117, 170
Anorexia, 55
Antibodies, 15, 17, 23, 28, 32, 33, 42, 43, 45, 49, 50, 51, 52, 63, 84, 101, 146, 166, 167, 181, 182
Anxiety, i, ii, 10, 22, 72, 73, 76, 97, 139, 172, 181, 204
Armour, 37, 39, 100, 116, 141, 142, 143, 144, 146, 148, 151, 156, 189
Autism, ii, 120
Autoimmune, iv, 11, 14, 16, 23, 42, 44, 52, 85, 110, 115, 117, 131, 134, 165, 172, 204, 215

B12, 44, 50, 77, 89, 168, 174, 179, 183, 186
BBT, 59, 60
Blood Pressure, 115, 116, 136, 150, 151, 159
Blood Sugar, 49, 52, 64, 74, 75, 80, 127, 128, 129, 160, 200
Blood Test, 12, 17, 32, 33, 37, 38, 41, 45, 52, 63, 68, 69, 72, 78, 98, 102, 104, 117, 134, 137, 141, 153, 154, 166, 168, 174, 190, 192, 207, 208, 213
Brain Fog, 10, 43, 46, 74, 79, 111, 121, 128, 131, 166, 169, 173, 183, 198

Caffeine, 49, 76, 84, 106, 113, 170
Cancer, 35, 59, 70, 216
Cervical Fluid, 55, 62
Coeliac, 45
Coffee, 40, 107
Congenital Hypothyroidism, ii, 14, 22, 25, 207
Constipation, 9, 104, 121, 173, 198

Conversion, 13, 37, 49
Cortisol, 49, 52, 58, 67, 72, 74, 76, 80, 83, 126, 128, 159, 204, 206
Cushing's, 74

Depression, 10, 22, 73, 76, 118, 139, 148, 172, 173, 181
Diet, 9, 44, 45, 66, 72, 75, 79, 80, 82, 106, 133, 138, 167, 178, 203
DIO2, 13
Disordered Eating, 49, 55, 67, 82, 205

Egg, 22, 53, 54, 55, 58, 65, 66, 79, 88
Endocrinologist, vi, 97, 101, 115, 120, 137, 143, 147, 152
Endometriosis, 57, 59, 62, 64, 89

Fatigue, 9, 10, 16, 43, 46, 60, 69, 72, 74, 84, 105, 111, 117, 121, 127, 130, 141, 148, 155, 166, 168, 171, 172, 183, 196, 198, 199
Ferritin, 64, 77, 154, 168, 174, 179, 183, 186
Fibroid, 57, 59, 64, 70
Flare, i, 27, 43, 67, 79, 85, 111, 113, 126, 127, 145, 149, 153, 167, 169, 176, 184, 196, 197, 201
Folic Acid, 49, 77, 78, 86, 89, 104
Free T3, 12, 14, 22, 23, 32, 33, 34, 36, 51, 82, 98, 99, 142, 147, 153, 182, 190
Free T4, 12, 13, 14, 22, 33, 34, 37, 98, 99, 101, 142, 151, 153, 182, 190
Full Thyroid Panel, 12, 32, 33, 38, 39, 57, 97, 98, 137, 154, 182

Gestational Diabetes, 115, 117, 129, 154
Gluten, 17, 44, 46, 76, 106, 112, 205
Goitrogenic, 47
Graves', 172

Gut, 14, 44, 50, 67, 70, 71, 75, 119, 167, 176, 187, 188, 203, 205

Hair Loss, 10, 63, 74, 168, 184
Hashimoto's, i, 11, 14, 15, 16, 23, 25, 42, 44, 49, 50, 51, 52, 59, 63, 65, 68, 71, 72, 76, 79, 84, 86, 101, 115, 130, 141, 144, 146, 152, 153, 155, 156, 165, 166, 168, 173, 183, 200, 204, 205, 215
HCG, 96, 99
Headaches, 49, 57, 79, 80, 116, 150, 168, 198
Heart Palpitations, 74, 117, 126, 172
Hyperthyroidism, 34, 43, 57, 59, 172, 190
Hypnobirthing, 129, 158, 159, 218

Intrahepatic Cholestasis, 144, 146, 149
Iodine, 104, 205
Iron, 40, 44, 50, 64, 77, 89, 104
Itchy, 10, 105, 144, 146

LDN, 52
Levothyroxine, 12, 13, 34, 37, 51, 100, 101, 102, 117, 137, 142, 146, 148, 151, 152, 189
Low Papp-A, 115, 149

Magnesium, 40, 49, 50, 70, 78, 104, 121
Mastitis, 189, 193
Medical Exemption Certificate, 98, 122
Menopause, 53, 204, 207
Migraines, 10, 49, 57, 60, 68, 69, 71, 95, 105, 111, 117, 154, 168, 198
Miscarriage, i, ii, 22, 23, 25, 28, 31, 32, 43, 53, 55, 66, 87, 100, 106, 116, 120, 143
MTHFR, 78

Obstetrician, vi, 37, 97, 115, 120, 139, 142, 144, 150, 151
Oestrogen, 40, 53, 54, 58, 68, 69, 70
Oestrogen Dominance, 49, 60, 61, 68, 69, 71, 72, 75
Omega 3, 78, 86, 89, 104
Optimal Levels, 12, 15, 22, 32, 33, 34, 41, 51, 87, 97, 98, 141, 155, 166, 190
Ovaries, 22, 23, 32, 54, 62, 63, 68
Ovulation, i, 22, 54, 55, 57, 59, 60, 61, 63, 65, 67, 69, 72, 96
Oxytocin, 158, 159

PCOS, 55, 57, 59, 61, 62, 115
Pelvic Floor, 178
Perimenopause, 53
Periods, i, 27, 53, 54, 56, 60, 63, 64, 67, 68, 69, 71, 78, 95, 112, 155
Pre-eclampsia, 22, 25, 86, 115, 116, 120, 150
Probiotic, 50, 71, 77, 89, 104
Progesterone, 53, 54, 58, 68, 69
Prolactin, 22, 190

Remission, 25, 26, 42, 72, 110, 141, 146, 155, 166, 167, 183

Selenium, 14, 17, 49, 50, 51, 77, 78, 89, 104
Self-sourced, 39, 116, 143
Sleep, 60, 66, 67, 72, 73, 75, 83, 107, 112, 119, 128, 166, 167, 168, 171, 176, 183, 198, 199, 206, 207
Soy, 45, 46, 205
Sperm, 22, 54, 55, 62, 66, 86
Spoon Theory, 85, 89, 208
Strength Training, 66, 108, 129, 175
Subclinical Hypothyroidism, 15, 23, 36, 62, 100, 116, 122

T3, 9, 12, 13, 22, 34, 36, 37, 38, 39, 51, 101, 102, 153, 182, 183, 220

T4, 9, 12, 13, 14, 18, 22, 34, 36, 37, 38, 51, 99, 101, 102, 117, 137, 146

TSH, 12, 13, 15, 22, 33, 34, 35, 62, 98, 143, 145, 182, 190

Vaccines, 109, 144, 149

Vitamin C, 50, 76, 77, 89, 104, 170

Vitamin D, 17, 50, 51, 77, 86, 104, 168, 174, 179, 183, 186, 205

Vitamin K2, 50, 104

Weight Loss, 66, 82, 172, 177, 191

Yoga, 11, 66, 75, 76, 108, 121, 122, 128, 131, 132, 170, 175, 201

Zinc, 14, 49, 50, 77, 78, 86, 104, 170

Appendix (References)

[1] https://pubmed.ncbi.nlm.nih.gov/19190113/
[2] https://drknews.com/unraveling-thyroid-antibodies/
[3] https://www.theinvisiblehypothyroidism.com/take-back-control-order-your-own-thyroid-tests/
[4] https://www.ncbi.nlm.nih.gov/pubmed/31808375
[5] https://www.liebertpub.com/doi/10.1089/thy.2014.0029
[6] https://www.healio.com/news/endocrinology/20180709/thyroid-function-antibody-positivity-associated-with-ovarian-reserve-in-infertility
[7] https://www.healio.com/news/endocrinology/20180709/thyroid-function-antibody-positivity-associated-with-ovarian-reserve-in-infertility
[8] https://cks.nice.org.uk/topics/hypothyroidism/management/overt-hypothyroidism-non-pregnant/
[9] https://www.btf-thyroid.org/Handlers/Download.ashx?IDMF=941f817e-a8da-4ea9-8ee9-83772477c280
[10] https://www.ncbi.nlm.nih.gov/pubmed/15705921/
[11] https://www.sciencedirect.com/science/article/pii/S2214623719301528
[12] http://www.aacc.org/sitecollectiondocuments/nacb/lmpg/thyroid/thyroid-fullversion.pdf
[13] https://www.ncbi.nlm.nih.gov/pubmed/11836274
[14] https://www.ncbi.nlm.nih.gov/pubmed/29396968
[15] https://www.oatext.com/the-definition-of-optimal-metabolism-and-its-association-with-large-reductions-in-chronic-diseases.php
[16] https://pubmed.ncbi.nlm.nih.gov/38635065/

[17] https://in.bgu.ac.il/en/fohs/communityhealth/Family/Documents/HYPOTHYROIDISM%20Guidelines%20ATA%20AACE%202012.pdf
[18] https://www.thyroidmanager.org/chapter/adult-hypothyroidism/#toc-9-8-1-pharmacology-of-thyroid-hormone-replacement-preparations1
[19] https://www.thyroidmanager.org/chapter/adult-hypothyroidism/#toc-9-8-1-pharmacology-of-thyroid-hormone-replacement-preparations1
[20] https://www.ncbi.nlm.nih.gov/pubmed/3066320
[21] https://www.ncbi.nlm.nih.gov/pubmed/31808375
[22] https://www.ncbi.nlm.nih.gov/pubmed/11932302
[23] https://www.ncbi.nlm.nih.gov/pubmed/27186560
[24] https://pubmed.ncbi.nlm.nih.gov/10468932/
[25] https://www.ncbi.nlm.nih.gov/pubmed/15012623
[26] https://www.ncbi.nlm.nih.gov/pubmed/15012623
[27] https://www.ncbi.nlm.nih.gov/pubmed/22115162
[28] https://www.ncbi.nlm.nih.gov/pubmed/20332127
[29] https://pubmed.ncbi.nlm.nih.gov/2371025/
[30] https://www.ncbi.nlm.nih.gov/pmc/articles/PMC2533153
[31] http://www.newswise.com/articles/mild-thyroid-dysfunction-in-early-pregnancy-linked-to-serious-complications
[32] https://www.liebertpub.com/doi/10.1089/thy.2014.0029
[33] https://cks.nice.org.uk/topics/hypothyroidism/management/preconception-or-pregnant/
[34] https://www.ncbi.nlm.nih.gov/pubmed/31808375
[35] https://www.nhs.uk/conditions/pregnancy-and-baby/foods-to-avoid-pregnant/
[36] https://www.nichd.nih.gov/health/topics/high-risk/conditioninfo/factors

[37] https://www.ncbi.nlm.nih.gov/pubmed/31808375
[38] https://www.thelancet.com/journals/landia/article/PIIS2213-8587(22)00007-9/fulltext
[39] https://www.thyroid.org/wp-content/uploads/publications/ctfp/volume7/issue1/ct_public_v71_3.pdf
[40] https://www.nhs.uk/Conditions/thyroiditis/Pages/Introduction.aspx#post-partum
[41] https://www.btf-thyroid.org/information/leaflets/38-pregnancy-and-fertility-guide
[42] https://www.ncbi.nlm.nih.gov/pubmed/22378092

www.ingramcontent.com/pod-product-compliance
Lightning Source LLC
Chambersburg PA
CBHW031146020426
42333CB00013B/539